501 EASY HEALTH TIPS

Published in 2007 by
New Holland Publishers (UK) Ltd
London • Cape Town • Sydney • Auckland
www.newhollandpublishers.com

Garfield House, 86–88 Edgware Road,
London W2 2EA, United Kingdom
80 McKenzie Street, Cape Town 8001, South Africa
Unit 4, 66 Gibbes Street, Chatswood,
NSW 2067, Australia
218 Lake Road, Northcote, Auckland, New Zealand

ISBN: 978 1 84537 676 5

Editor: Anne Konopelski
Editorial Direction: Rosemary Wilkinson
Production: Hazel Kirkman
Design: Paul Wright
Artwork: Paul Wright

10 9 8 7 6 5 4 3 2

Reproduction by Modern Age Repro house Ltd,
Hong Kong
Printed and bound by Craft Print International,
Singapore

Disclaimer
The author and publishers have made every effort
to ensure that all information given in this book is
safe and accurate, but they cannot accept liability
for any resulting injury or loss or damage to either
property or person, whether direct or consequential
or however arising.

Abbreviations
The following abbreviations are used throughout
the book:

cm	centimetre
fl oz	fluid ounce
g	gram
in	inch
kg	kilogram
lb	pound
mg	millligram
ml	millilitre
oz	ounce
tsp	teaspoon
Tbsp	Tablespoon

501 EASY HEALTH TIPS

KELLIE COLLINS

NEW
HOLLAND

Introduction

There are various definitions for health, including 'the absence of disease' or 'physical, mental and social well-being' – but my favourite is 'a toast or a wish for someone's well-being'. I can't prevent disease or cure illness, but I hope that by reading this book, you will be able to take small steps towards changing your health for the better. You certainly don't have to take on all 501 tips. There are some that won't apply to you, and I would never expect anyone to start cycling, swimming and going to the gym all in one day. All in the one lifetime, even!

When I tell people I'm a nutritionist, most automatically assume I'm a health freak. Okay, so I do eat a healthy diet most of the time but I am also partial to a glass of wine and a bar of chocolate. I don't see the point in denying myself these things as long as I have them in moderation (the 80:20 rule, if you like – tip 223).

I'm a foodie and I believe that everything I eat has got to be worth eating. There's no point in wasting good eating time with rubbish food. So I hope you'll be inspired to go back to basics in the Food and Drink chapter and cook some meals from scratch. You'll see that it doesn't take all day or a cupboard full of ingredients to put together something really tasty.

I'm not a big fan of the word 'diet'. People find it off-putting, and it conjures up images of something short-term. Healthy eating should be something you take on for life. You'll see in the Weight Loss chapter that I try to use the D-word as little as possible, preferring instead to use terms like 'way of eating'. After all, the general definition for diet is 'what a person eats and drinks'. No mention there of weight loss or something you do to fit into a new dress! The safest and most effective way to achieve weight loss is to eat healthily, control your portions and exercise.

Which brings me to the Fitness chapter – I don't want anyone to sneakily skip over it! I used to be a fully paid-up member of the 'I hate exercise' club, complete with self-diagnosed gym phobia. Eventually the messages I was preaching on a daily basis about the importance of exercise – not only for weight loss, but for general health – started to filter into my own mind. I suppose I was curious to see what all the fuss was about. Could sweating and panting for an hour on a treadmill really make you feel good afterwards? Is exercise really one of the best ways to relieve stress? And as much as I hate to admit it, the answer to both questions is yes. Have a look through the chapter and see. You'll probably be surprised at how easy it can be to introduce

exercise into your lifestyle. You can even get fit in front of the television if you put your mind to it.

In fact, I'm willing to bet that you'll be surprised at how easy it is to improve your overall health by making a few small changes to your lifestyle – gradually. As you'll see by the time you reach the end of this book, being healthy is easy when you know how!

Kellie Collins

FOOD AND DRINK

1. WHAT'S COOKING?

Forget additive-loaded, processed foods and ready meals. Make your own meals from scratch so you know exactly what's in them. You don't have to be a gourmet chef to succeed. Start with some key, basic dishes, and the world of ingredients will be your oyster.

2. SAFETY FIRST

Prevent food poisoning in your kitchen by keeping raw and cooked meats separate. Store raw meat below cooked meat in the refrigerator and use separate chopping boards and knives for each. Always wash your hands after handling raw meat. Store leftovers in the fridge and discard them after two days.

3. FREEZE FRAME

Freezing food is an economical and time-saving way of keeping it safe. Put frozen food from the supermarket into your freezer as soon as possible. Wait until leftovers and cooked foods are cold before freezing them. (Placing warm foods in the freezer will raise its overall temperature.) Wrap food for freezing carefully to prevent freezer burn and cross-contamination. Defrost food thoroughly before using and never refreeze it.

4. GREAT GRAINS

Wholegrains are grain foods in which all parts of the grain are intact and retained during any processing. Wholemeal also contains all parts of the grain but is milled to a finer texture. Wholegrain has a lower GI (see tip 166), but both are good choices and should be chosen over white flour products, which have 66 per cent less fibre.

5. BREAD OF LIFE

Vary your bread choice – try rye, bagels, ciabatta, tortillas or potato bread for a change from the sliced loaf. Bread is a low-fat staple food for many people and a good source of carbohydrates. There are many different types of bread, and those made with wholemeal or wholegrain flours are generally a better option than those made with white flour.

6. GOING CRACKERS

Crackers are a good alternative to bread – especially wheat-free crackers, which suit anyone who suffers from wheat intolerance. Oatcakes are high in fibre and delicious served with hummus or cheese, or as an accompaniment to soup. Rice cakes are gluten free; serve them with cottage cheese and chopped tomato for a healthy snack.

7. SPREADING OUT

When choosing a spread for your bread, check the label and make sure it is low in trans fats (see tip 132). Trans fats are formed when liquid oils are converted to solid spreads and have been linked to heart disease. Use olive or sunflower spreads instead of butter and vegetable margarine, both of which are high in trans fats.

8. CEREAL-OUSLY SIMPLE

Cereal with milk is the ultimate convenience food, and a meal in itself. Eaten any time of day, but especially for breakfast, high-fibre cereals fill you up and boost your energy levels. Many cereals are fortified with vitamins and minerals, increasing their nutritional values. Avoid sugar-coated cereals and compare sugar contents of mueslis to choose the low-sugar varieties.

9. OAT SO GOOD

Oats are rich in soluble and insoluble fibres, B vitamins and protein. They're naturally low in sugar, fat and salt, and have been shown to reduce levels of LDL (bad) cholesterol. Oats are also low GI (see tip 166), so try to include them in your diet at every opportunity.

10. BACK TO PORRIDGE

Here are a few easy ways to incorporate oats into your diet:
- Have porridge for breakfast. Add dried fruit, honey, nuts and seeds for extra flavour and goodness.
- Make your own muesli or buy varieties with no added sugar.
- Add some oats to fruit crumble toppings.
- Add oats to smoothies for extra creaminess. Soak them in milk overnight and combine with fruit and yoghurt the next morning.

11. HOME-MADE MUESLI

Put 200g (7oz) porridge oats, 25g (1oz) wheatgerm, 50g (1¾oz) barley flakes and 25g (1oz) each of hazelnuts and pumpkin seeds on a baking tray. Toast them in the oven for 10 minutes at 150°C (300°F/Gas mark 2), shaking the tray halfway through. Allow the seeds to cool and mix in 150g (5½oz) dried fruit such as apricots, cranberries and sultanas. This can be stored in an airtight jar for two weeks. Serve with milk.

12. BEST BREAKFASTS

- porridge made with semi-skimmed milk and topped with some banana slices or raisins
- boiled or scrambled eggs with wholegrain toast and orange juice
- oatcakes spread with peanut butter or high-fruit jam
- lean, grilled bacon with some grilled tomato and a toasted granary roll
- mixed fruit salad topped with Greek yoghurt and some chopped nuts

13. SAY CHEESE

Cheese is often cited as a good source of protein, but it contributes considerably to fat intake. Even low-fat cheeses can still contain up to half of their calories as fat, so compare labels and check saturated fat and sodium contents. Get your protein from other sources whenever possible (see tip 135).

14. CHEESY BITES

Choose stronger-tasting cheeses and you'll use less, reducing fat intake and calories. Add feta to salads, melt goat's cheese over vegetables and stir mozzarella into pasta.

15. IN THE DARK

Include dark green leaves in your summer salads. These contain more nutrients, such as beta carotene and fibre, than paler leaves. Try watercress, rocket, lamb's lettuce or radicchio.

16. THE PERFECT CATCH

Try to eat at least two portions of fish each week, including one portion of oily fish. Oily fish such as salmon, mackerel, trout and sardines have more Omega 3 fatty acids (see tip 131) than white fish. Pregnant women should eat no more than two portions of oily fish each week, however, as toxins may build up in the flesh of the fish.

17. EASY SALMON FISH CAKES

Drain 120g (4oz) tinned salmon and mix with 120g (4oz) mashed potatoes. Beat a large egg and add half to the mixture. Add 2 tsp curry powder, a pinch of salt and pepper, and a squeeze of lemon juice to taste. Shape the mixture into four fish cakes and coat each with the rest of the beaten egg. Give each fish cake a light dusting of plain flour and coat with some wholegrain breadcrumbs. Bake in an oven at 180°C (350°F/Gas mark 4) for 20 minutes, then serve immediately.

18. FISH TALES
Dip prawns in chilli sauce or add them to stir-fries. Add tinned, drained tuna to pasta or marinade salmon in teriyaki sauce and fry.

19. FISH FOOD
Check out the catch at your local fishmonger and have fun trying out different types like red snapper, squid, sea bass, monkfish and sole.

20. STEAMY WINDOWS
Research has shown that fresh broccoli loses up to 97 per cent of its key antioxidants when it is boiled, but just 11 per cent if it is steamed for 5 minutes. If you notice other vegetables losing colour during cooking, that means they're losing nutrients, too.

21. HIDE AND LEEK
If you're having trouble persuading your kids to try eating different vegetables, add finely chopped or grated vegetables like carrots and courgettes to stews, pasta sauces, meatballs or cottage pie. Your kids won't even know they're eating vegetables! Also try mashing a little parsnip or cauliflower into potatoes, perhaps with a little low-fat, grated cheddar.

22. PERFECT POMEGRANATE

Pomegranate juice is bursting with vitamins A, C, E and folic acid, giving it three times more antioxidant power than green tea or red wine. Recent studies have shown that pomegranate juice may reduce bad (LDL) cholesterol levels and your risk of heart disease, osteoarthritis and some cancers.

23. POMEGRANATE MOCKTAIL

Add one star anise and one cinnamon stick to 600ml (20fl oz) pomegranate juice. Set aside for a few hours or overnight. Just before serving, whizz 150g (5½oz) of an assortment of berries in a blender, keeping a few aside. Add some crushed ice to four tall glasses with the leftover berries, then add the crushed berries and pomegranate juice. Serve immediately.

24. ZEST IS BEST

Citrus peel is packed with flavour and vitamin C, so don't waste it. Grate lemon or lime zest into chicken and fish dishes, soups, salads or rice. Add it to black or green tea and drinking water for a tangy flavour. Before grating the fruit, be sure to wash and dry it thoroughly.

25. CUT DOWN ON CAFFEINE

A high caffeine intake is linked to several health problems, including osteoporosis and high blood pressure. Instant coffee contains up to 70mg of caffeine per cup, so switch to decaffeinated coffee or rooibos tea, which is caffeine free.

26. TEA FOR TWO

Black and green teas contain anti-ageing antioxidants. Drinking tea may also improve your memory and reduce your risk of stroke, heart disease and some cancers. Swap some of your daily cups of coffee each day for tea. It still contains caffeine, but less than coffee.

27. FRY LIGHT

Always grill foods when possible and avoid deep frying. If you really must fry your food, however, use olive oil. It is more stable at high temperatures than butter and so retains most of its nutritional benefits, such as essential fatty acids (see tip 131). Butter is high in unhealthy saturated fats (see tip 133), and its instability at high temperatures may affect the flavour of your dishes.

28. COOKING UNDER PRESSURE

If your pressure cooker hasn't seen the light of day since the 80s, dust it down and rediscover its advantages. The quick cooking times are more economical and lock in flavour and nutrients, making more delicious and nutritious meals. Pressure cookers are especially good for cooking cheaper cuts of meat, soups and casseroles.

29. PASSION BOOSTERS

Shellfish, pumpkin seeds, pine nuts, wholegrains and pulses all contain zinc, which is required for the production of testosterone – a hormone that regulates sex drive in men and women.

30. GET FRIENDLY WITH BACTERIA

Try to include probiotics and prebiotics in your everyday diet. This won't be difficult, as they are now added to many foods, such as yoghurts, milk and breakfast cereals. The following are some of the reported health benefits of eating these friendly bacteria:

- lowering of blood pressure and blood cholesterol
- replacement of beneficial bacteria after a course of antibiotics
- prevention of candida

31. VARIETY IS THE SPICE OF LIFE

Don't be afraid to experiment when you are cooking or eating out and try as many new foods as your taste buds dare. Research has shown that eating a wide variety of foods (typically 27 different foods every day) is associated with a greater life expectancy.

32. NO MORE NAUSEA

Morning sickness, motion sickness and sometimes even hangover sickness (depending on the extent!) may all be relieved by sipping ginger tea. It can also help alleviate colds and release trapped wind.

33. NOT A GRAIN OF TRUTH

People who buy rock or sea salt mistakenly believe it's better for them. All types of salt contain the same amount of sodium, and since most of our salt intake comes hidden in foods, it's best to avoid adding extra salt to food during cooking or at the table.

34. CHOOSE LOW-SALT FOODS

The bulk of our salt intake comes from purchased bread, breakfast cereals, soups, sauces, ready meals and even biscuits. With all this salt hidden in our food, check the nutritional information on the packaging and choose items with the lowest salt content. As a general guide, 1.25g of salt or 0.5g of sodium per 100g is a lot of salt, and 0.25g of salt or 0.1g of sodium per 100g is a small amount of salt.

35. TOP TIPS TO REDUCE SALT INTAKE

- Aim for an intake of 6g (⅙oz) salt or less each day.
- Season your food with herbs and spices instead of salt during cooking.
- Don't automatically add salt at the table – taste your food first.
- Cut down on your intake of ready meals.
- Buy fresh produce rather than tinned fruit and vegetables.
- Read the labels and compare the salt content of similar foods (see tip 34).

36. TAKE FIVE A DAY

Eat at least five portions of fruit and vegetables each day. One portion of fruit is approximately 80g (3oz), or any of the following:

- one apple, banana, pear, orange or other fruit of a similar size
- two plums, mandarins, kiwi fruits or satsumas
- one slice of a large fruit such as a melon or a pineapple
- 3 Tbsp fruit salad in natural juice
- 1 Tbsp dried fruit
- 15 grapes, cherries or berries

37. VEGGIN' OUT

One portion of vegetables is approximately 80g (3oz), or any of the following:

- a small bowl of salad
- 3 heaped Tbsp vegetables (raw or cooked)
- half a pepper
- four broccoli florets
- three celery sticks
- seven cherry tomatoes

38. JUICE IT UP

Invest in a juicer and start the day with a refreshing, healthy drink. Bear in mind that no matter how much juice you drink in a day, it still only counts as one portion of fruit because fibre and other nutrients are lost during the juicing process. Still, drinking fresh, home-made juice is a great way to stock up on immunity-boosting vitamin C.

39. JUICY FRUITS

- Juice one apple, four carrots, two kiwi fruits and one thumb-sized piece of fresh, peeled ginger.
- Juice one peeled beetroot, three carrots, two pears, one peeled lime and five torn basil leaves.
- Juice a whole cucumber, two celery sticks and two apples.

40. SMOOTH TALKIN'

Smoothies are filling, easy to digest and perfect for a quick energy boost. Because the whole fruit is used, you get all the goodness. If you're buying a ready-made smoothie, check the ingredients for high-calorie items such as cream, full-fat yoghurt and honey. It's easy to make your own smoothies at home with a hand-held blender, some fruit and crushed ice.

41. GO BANANAS!

Bananas are the ultimate snack food. They'll boost your energy instantly, as well as raising your potassium levels. (Potassium is essential for regulating your nerves, heartbeat and blood pressure.) Bananas can also be useful hangover cures after a big night out on the town.

42. BERRY WELL

Berries are packed with fibre and vitamin C, and are a great addition to cereal, yoghurt or fruit salad. Keep bags of frozen berries in the freezer for a sweet treat. A 100g (3½oz) serving of strawberries has 77mg of vitamin C. That's twice as much vitamin C than you'll get from the same serving of grapefruit.

43. BANANA BERRY SMOOTHIE

Blend one small ripe banana with 3 Tbsp mixed berries (strawberries, raspberries or whatever's in season) and 200ml (7fl oz) semi-skimmed milk. Add some crushed ice and blend until smooth. Serves one.

44. WORKING LUNCH

- Seeded breads and rolls are low GI and will keep your energy levels up for longer. Buy them in packs of four or six and freeze. Defrost them overnight before using.
- Mix leftover cooked pasta with chopped tomatoes, cucumber, cheese, cooked meat or fish and salad dressing.
- Dip carrot and celery sticks into hummus or cream cheese.
- Chop up kiwi fruits, melon slices, apples, oranges and grapes, and pop in a lunchbox for a great fruit salad.

45. CALMING CAMOMILE

Camomile tea contains a compound called apigenin. This works on the same part of your brain as anti-anxiety drugs, so it's great for helping with relaxation and lowering stress levels. A cup before bedtime will help you sleep better.

46. BLUEBERRY HILL

Blueberries are one of the healthiest foods you can eat. Their blue colour comes from powerful plant pigments called anthocyanins, which have 2,400 times the antioxidant power of vitamin E (itself considered a powerful antioxidant). Add blueberries to smoothies, fruit salads and cereals, and use in baking.

47. TUNE YOUR TASTE BUDS

Once you start eating wholegrain bread instead of white, and omitting added salt from your food, it will become second nature. Eventually you'll find that the old foods don't appeal anymore, and any added salt will make your food taste horrible!

48. SWEET SURRENDER

The ingredients list of a food always starts with the ingredients that are contained in the greatest quantities. If sugar or anything ending in 'ose' is high up on the list, it's probably best to avoid the food. Check the sugar content on the nutrition panel. As a general rule, 10g (¼oz) or more of sugar per 100g (3½oz) is a lot of sugar, whereas 2g or less per 100g (3½oz) is a small amount of sugar.

49. READ THE LABEL

Pay attention to the fat and saturated fat content of foods by reading the nutritional information on their labels. Twenty grams (¾oz) or more of fat, and 5g (⅙oz) or more of saturated fat, per 100g (3½oz) is a lot of fat. Three grams (⅙oz) or less of fat, and 1g or less of saturates, is a little fat.

50. GRAB A LOW GI BREAKFAST

For a low GI breakfast that will fill you up and keep you going for longer, swap orange juice and toasted white bread with jam for toasted granary bread topped with banana slices or a yoghurt and berry smoothie.

51. TOP TEN FOODS TO AVOID

- doughnuts
- sugar-coated breakfast cereals
- soft drinks
- sausage rolls
- jelly beans
- Danish pastries
- bacon
- hot dogs
- potato crisps
- pork pies

52. VEGGIE VOGUE

Vegetarian and vegan diets don't have to be restrictive. Eating plenty of plant foods, including fruit, vegetables, pulses, beans, grains, nuts and seeds; low-fat dairy or soya products; and low-fat vegetable oils such as olive oil, will ensure you are getting a good balance of nutrients.

53. TOP UP WITH TOMATOES

Tomatoes are an excellent source of vitamin C and the antioxidant lycopene, which may help prevent prostate cancer. Lycopene becomes even more potent when cooked, so choose tomato-based sauces and add tomato purée or ketchup to dishes – Shepherd's pie or spaghetti Bolognese, for example – while they're cooking.

54. TOMATO BRUSCHETTA

Halve eight cherry tomatoes and marinate for 30 minutes with one crushed garlic clove, four torn basil leaves and 1 Tbsp olive oil. Lightly toast four slices of crusty French bread under a grill. Remove, then top each slice with some of the tomato mixture. Heat under the grill for 2 minutes, then serve with the garlic and basil oil drizzled over. Serves two as a starter or snack.

55. EAT YOUR GREENS

Broccoli is packed with folate, vitamin C, beta carotene, potassium and a phytochemical called sulphoraphane, which helps reduce your risk of cancer. If you can't face a big pile of broccoli on the side of your plate, mix it into pasta sauce, add it to stir-fries or even have it raw in salads.

56. HONEY-ROASTED VEGETABLES

Chop one red pepper, two courgettes, one aubergine and one red onion into 5-cm (2-in) pieces. Halve eight cherry tomatoes and place all the vegetables in a bowl. In a small cup, mix 2 tsp honey, 1 Tbsp olive oil and one crushed garlic clove. Add the mixture to the vegetables and blend well. Spread out the vegetables on a baking tray and roast in the oven for 30 minutes at 180°C (350°F/Gas mark 4). Serve as a side dish or with rice.

57. FRESH OR FROZEN?

Some nutrients are lost during transport and storage of fresh vegetables, so you never really know how nutritious they are. However, freezing vegetables straight after they have been harvested preserves their nutrient content at the highest levels – so don't feel guilty about reaching for frozen vegetables if all that's left in the greengrocer are some bendy carrots.

58. RAISE THE STEAKS

Red meat is a great source of zinc, vitamin B12 and iron. Choose lean cuts and avoid cheap products such as burgers and pies, which are very high in saturated fat. Try not to eat red meat more than three times a week. Use herbs rather than salt to season it, as salt will draw out moisture and make the finished dish dry.

59. BBQ BASICS

When you use the barbecue, make sure the coals are white hot before you cook your food. Ensure that all meat is cooked through before serving. Keep raw and cooked meats separate, and use different utensils for each. For a good vegetarian option, thread skewers with chunks of pepper, onion, mushroom and halloumi cheese, and grill.

60. PASS THE BUCK

Despite its name, buckwheat is gluten and wheat free, and makes an excellent alternative to pasta. It is traditionally used in pancakes, so even if you've never heard of it, you may have had it in a Chinese restaurant with crispy duck. Buckwheat can also be used in baking and is a good source of carbohydrates, protein, iron and calcium.

61. DON'T GIVE A FIG

Figs are an excellent source of fibre and calcium. If you can't get fresh figs, try dried ones; they're good as a snack when you are craving sugary foods. Fig purée – 200g (7oz) figs puréed with around 50–100ml (2–3½fl oz) of water or fruit juice – can also be used as a sweetener and as a fat substitute in baked goods.

62. BEET IT

Beetroot has made a comeback and is being hailed as a new superfood. It is packed with fibre, antioxidant vitamins including folate and minerals such as calcium. Pickled, boiled or roasted, enjoy beets in salads, soups and even cake (think carrot cake except with beetroot!).

63. GOOD NEWS FOR CHOCOLATE LOVERS

- Chocolate contains antioxidants that may protect against heart disease and cancer.
- A bar of milk chocolate provides around 15 per cent of your daily calcium requirements.
- Eaten after a meal, chocolate is less likely to cause tooth decay than other sweets.
- Although chocolate is one of the most craved foods, it's not addictive!

64. AND THE NOT SO GOOD NEWS...

A bar of chocolate provides 22 per cent of your daily fat intake, with most of that being saturated fat. The same bar will set you back approximately 300 calories, so if you absolutely must have chocolate every day, chop a bar into two or three pieces and eat one piece each day.

65. BEANS, BEANS THE MORE YOU EAT...

Baked beans are cheap, easy to cook and packed full of fibre. Made from haricot beans, they count towards your vegetable intake. (However, no matter how many you eat in one day, they still only count as one portion, because baked beans are higher in calories and carbohydrates than other vegetables, and the sauce can be high in salt and sugar.) The tomato sauce is also a rich source of the cancer-fighting compound lycopene.

66. CREAMY HERB PASTA

For a light, low-fat meal, mix some light cream cheese with cooked pasta. Add a handful of chopped, sundried tomatoes, some torn basil leaves and a squeeze of lemon juice to taste. Finish with a twist of freshly ground black pepper and serve immediately.

67. TURNING IN

Going to bed on a full stomach can trigger heartburn, which in turn causes insomnia. If you have no choice but to eat a late meal, have small portions and avoid spicy, fatty, garlicky foods. A cup of peppermint tea afterwards will aid digestion.

68. NUTTY FACTS

Although they are high in fat and calories, nuts are low in saturated fat – and most nuts, especially hazelnuts and macadamias, are also high in monounsaturates (see tip 134). All nuts are low GI and contain significant amounts of iron, zinc and magnesium, with Brazil nuts being particularly rich in selenium.

69. SOWING THE SEEDS

Handy snacks, sunflower, sesame, poppy and pumpkin seeds are rich in polyunsaturated fats, protein and minerals such as potassium, copper, zinc and magnesium. Add seeds to soups, salads, cereal and yoghurt for extra crunch.

70. THE ULTIMATE COMFORT FOOD?

Cheap and cheerful, whether boiled, baked or mashed, potatoes never fail to fill you up. They're packed full of vitamin C and lots of other vitamins and minerals. Eat the skin of baked potatoes for the fibre and go easy on the chips!

71. KEEP THE VAMPIRES AWAY

Garlic has anti-cancer compounds and cholesterol-lowering, antibacterial and decongestant properties. Add it to practically any savoury dish during cooking or, if you're not mad about the taste (or smell), pop a whole clove of garlic in the oven while you're cooking a pizza. Soft and spreadable like butter, roast garlic has a mellow flavour.

72. AMAZING AVOCADO

Avocados are rich in heart-healthy monounsaturated fat, vitamin E and other vitamins and minerals. Add half a chopped avocado to your salad or make guacamole for a delicious dip. Using avocado oil in salads helps your body absorb the antioxidants from peppers and tomatoes.

73. CREAMY GUACAMOLE

Mix together one diced, ripe avocado, two chopped tomatoes, two minced garlic cloves, 2 Tbsp fresh, chopped coriander, 1 Tbsp Greek yoghurt and 1 Tbsp fresh lime juice. Season with salt and freshly ground black pepper. Serve as a dip with vegetable sticks or with burgers, as an alternative to ketchup.

74. PITTA CHIPS

Replace high-fat, high-salt crisps and tortilla chips with wedge-shaped slices of pitta bread or flour tortillas. Cut two pittas into wedges and bake them in the oven for 10–15 minutes at 180°C (350°F/Gas mark 4). Remove from the oven and sprinkle with a little paprika or cayenne pepper for extra flavour. Serves two as a side dish or for dipping.

75. FIERY FAJITAS

This is a quick, low-fat dish, rich in antioxidants thanks to the peppers, guacamole and tomatoes. Stir-fry two chopped chicken fillets, one chopped red pepper and one small, chopped onion. Add a packet of fajita spice mix. Warm two large flour tortillas, then fill with the chicken mix. Serve with guacamole, salsa and grated low-fat cheese.

76. BROWNED OFF

Unlike white rice, brown rice is not processed and therefore retains its abundance of B vitamins and fibre. Brown rice is also low in fat, making it an ideal complex carbohydrate. It is especially good for anyone with gluten or wheat intolerance, or anyone following a low GI diet.

77. BALSAMIC BERRIES

Balsamic vinegar contains anti-ageing antioxidants and is also thought to aid digestion. Mix balsamic vinegar with olive oil for a delicious dressing that can be added to soups and stir-fries, and sprinkled over baked potatoes instead of butter or sour cream. Serve strawberries with a dash of balsamic vinegar for a delectable dessert.

78. GRAB A LOW GI LUNCH

Swap a ham and cheese sandwich on white bread for skinless chicken on a wholemeal pitta, served with a salad. Alternatively, replace a baked potato topped with cheese with lentil soup, served with a granary roll and cottage cheese.

79. LEAN CUISINE

Choose lean cuts of meat and always trim away any excess fat before grilling, not frying, it. Remove the skin from chicken and turkey, and don't eat the fat on bacon, no matter how tempting it is!

80. ON THE CONTINENT

Eating a Mediterranean-style diet could extend your life by up to one year. It will also reduce your risk of stroke, heart disease and cancer. Eat less red meat and include olive oil, fish, vegetables, nuts, seeds and grains in your diet. Oh, and the odd glass of red wine won't hurt.

81. BULK UP WITH BULGUR

A type of wheat, bulgur is a versatile grain that can be bought in a ready-to-use form, similar to couscous. It can be eaten hot, as an alternative to rice, pasta or potatoes, or cold in salads such as tabbouleh. Bulgur is high in fibre and a good source of B vitamins.

82. MEDITERRANEAN CHICKEN WITH BULGUR WHEAT

Cover 50g (1¾ oz) bulgur wheat with boiling water and leave for 15 minutes. Drain and mix with 4 chopped sun-dried tomatoes, 1 Tbsp pine nuts, 2 tsp capers, four chopped black olives and the juice of half a lemon. Serve with two grilled, sliced chicken fillets and a salad of cherry tomatoes and rocket. Serves two.

83. OUST THE LAGER LOUT

Beer contains phytochemicals that aid digestion and may help prevent heart disease. Remember that these effects are only seen in moderate drinkers – those who drink no more than two units (1 pint of beer) a day.

84. MILKING IT

Milk is one of the most nutritionally complete foods available. It is also naturally low in fat. Whole milk contains 4 per cent fat, and semi-skimmed milk contains 1.7 per cent fat. This means that a 200-ml (7-fl oz) glass of whole or semi-skimmed milk contains less fat than a packet of crisps or a regular-sized chocolate bar.

85. ADDING MILK TO YOUR DAILY DIET

- Try milky drinks like cocoa and lattes.
- Have cereal with milk for breakfast or supper.
- Use recipes with milk-based sauces, such as lasagne or fish pie.
- Add a small amount of milk to soup.
- Treat yourself to a few squares of milk chocolate.
- Try a milk-based dessert like rice pudding.

86. MILK ALTERNATIVES

For anyone who is lactose intolerant, or simply doesn't like the taste of milk, there are a number of alternatives. Soya milk, rice milk and oat milk are all available fortified with calcium and sweetened, flavoured or unsweetened. They are all good for drinking, putting on cereal and in cooking.

87. GET KEEN ON QUINOA

Pronounced keen-wa, this South American grain is a fantastic alternative to rice and pasta. Quinoa has a mild taste and a firm but slightly chewy texture. Its 14 per cent protein content makes it ideal for vegetarians, and its gluten-free properties means it is suitable for people with coeliac disease.

88. WILD ABOUT RICE

Wild rice isn't actually rice, but a type of grass. It is cooked and served the same way as other rices but takes about 50 minutes to prepare. Wild rice's subtle, nutty flavour enhances any dish and it provides protein, B vitamins, calcium and lots of fibre.

89. GRAB A LOW GI DINNER

Swap sausages and mash for grilled salmon with baked sweet potato and broccoli. Exchange pasta carbonara for pasta arrabiata and save on calories – and fat, too! Adding vegetables and salad to any meal will lower its overall GI value.

90. MAKE A BEELINE FOR HONEY

Use honey to sweeten smoothies and porridge, or have a small amount on wholegrain toast. Its healing properties have long been recognized. In fact, so great are honey's antibacterial and antifungal powers, it can be incorporated into wound dressings! A diet rich in honey also helps you build resistance to pollen and beat hay fever.

91. BETTER BAKING

Replace sugar in recipes with half the amount of honey or half dried fruit and half fruit juice. Save even more calories and fat by replacing half the fat in the recipe with bananas or yoghurt. Use wholemeal flour instead of white when baking bread, scones and muffins.

92. BLOTTING PAPER

Use paper towels or a napkin to soak up extra grease from fried foods, pizza or burgers when you are eating at home or dining out. You could easily soak up a teaspoon of grease, saving yourself 5g (⅙oz) fat and 50 calories.

93. RABBIT FOOD?

Salad doesn't have to mean limp lettuce leaves and squashed tomatoes. Use different varieties of crisp lettuce, cherry tomatoes, cucumber, grated carrot, raw broccoli, peppers and salad onions. Add feta, beans, egg, tuna or chicken for protein, and experiment by adding dried or fresh fruit. Slices of orange make a good topping.

94. PASS THE PARSLEY

Use fresh parsley in soups, salads, stir-fries and juices for its calming and breath-freshening properties. Parsley can also improve kidney and thyroid function, and aid digestion, so treat it as an ingredient in its own right and not simply as a garnish.

95. HERBAL REMEDY

Chop up leftover herbs, put them in an ice-cube tray with a little water and freeze them. When you need them, take the ice cubes straight from the freezer and add to dishes during cooking. Leftover wine (if there is such a thing!) can be treated in the same way.

96. CABBAGE PATCH

Don't boil cabbage to a grey sludge! Steam or lightly boil it just long enough to soften the leaves for a delicious, nutritious addition to mashed potatoes. Rich in folic acid, iron, vitamin C and anti-cancer agents, cabbage is also an essential component of any stir-fry.

97. BEAN ME UP

Make the most of beans and legumes; they are low GI and packed with fibre. Choose tinned varieties or, if you must use dried, make sure you soak them overnight, boil them in fresh water for 10 minutes, then simmer for 2–3 hours before cooking or serving.

98. TO BEAN OR NOT TO BEAN

Here are some easy ways of incorporating beans into your diet:

- Add beans or chick-peas to salads.
- Stir extra beans into soups, casseroles and sauces.
- Snack on hummus and crackers rather than cheese and crackers.
- Use lentils in dishes that call for minced meat.
- Spread a tortilla with refried beans before adding your fajita filling.
- Add kidney or black-eyed beans to chilli.

99. TUNA AND BEAN SALAD

Drain a tin of mixed beans and a tin of tuna, and combine. Add half a chopped red pepper, a quarter of a chopped red onion and some chopped parsley and basil, to taste. Drizzle with 1 Tbsp olive oil and 1 Tbsp balsamic vinegar. Serve with mixed leaves and cherry tomatoes. Serves two as a light lunch.

100. RHUBARB, RHUBARB

Stewed rhubarb is delicious served with thick, creamy yoghurt. If you suffer from constipation, rhubarb will get things moving. It stimulates the gut and is a rich source of vitamin C and fibre. Rhubarb also contains potassium and is low in sodium, making it excellent for the heart. Don't eat rhubarb leaves, though, as they are poisonous.

101. RHUBARB FOOL

Put 350g (12oz) rhubarb in a saucepan with 55g (2oz) sugar and the juice of an orange. Add enough water to cover the rhubarb and boil until it is soft. Whip one egg white until it is stiff and fold it into 50ml (2fl oz) whipped cream and 100ml (3½fl oz) Greek yoghurt. Fold the cooled rhubarb into the cream mixture, then serve immediately in four tall glasses.

102. PEAR SHAPED

Pears are a refreshing, low GI fruit and can be enjoyed on their own or in sweet or savoury dishes. Serve them in salads or with some crumbly feta or goat's cheese and walnuts. Alternatively, add them to apple crumble or bake them in the oven for a delicious dessert.

103. DRYING OUT
Dried fruit is high GI owing to its high sugar content, but it still contains valuable nutrients. Snack on dried fruits like apricots, raisins, figs or apples to satisfy a sweet craving. (Beware of banana chips, however, which usually have added honey.) Always try to choose dried fruits with no added sugar or honey.

104. KEEP IT LOCAL
Be aware of food miles – the distance your food has travelled before it reaches your plate. They can add up to the thousands for a simple salad or sandwich. Look out for farmers' markets in your area for fresh local produce and visit your local butcher instead of buying from the meat counter at the supermarket.

105. PEANUT BUTTER
Peanut butter doesn't actually contain butter – and, although it is high in fat, the peanuts are a good source of heart-healthy monounsaturates (see tip 134). Peanut butter makes a great addition to sauces, especially curries, and is delicious on toast for a filling snack. Look for sugar-free and low-fat varieties.

106. ONE EGG OR TWO?
Eggs are an excellent source of protein and iron, but the yolks are high in cholesterol and fat. If a recipe calls for two eggs, save on calories and fat by adding a whole egg and one egg white. People with high cholesterol should limit their intake of whole eggs to four each week. Healthy people can have up to seven eggs each week.

107. JAZZY EGGS

- Add some chopped, de-seeded tomatoes to cooked scrambled eggs.
- Make an omelette with sliced, leftover potatoes, some onion, peppers and beaten eggs.
- Halve cold boiled eggs, carefully remove the yolks, mash them with some mayonnaise, paprika and mustard, and use the mixture to stuff the egg whites.

108. DRESS IT UP

Use mustard, horseradish or pickle on your sandwiches instead of butter or spreads. You'll save calories and fat, and boost flavour. Tomato-based relishes are particularly good on ham and cheese sandwiches.

109. HYDRATION HABIT

You've heard it before, but it's very important that you drink at least eight glasses of water (each containing 200 ml/7fl oz) every day. Even mild dehydration will make you feel dizzy, weak and prone to headaches. Drinking pure water is the best way to rehydrate (tap water is fine), but unsweetened herbal teas will do the trick as well.

110. SOFT IN THE HEAD

Diet soft drinks contain a variety of artificial sweeteners that are safe in moderation. They also contain a raft of other artificial ingredients and phosphorus, however – which, if not balanced by a good intake of calcium, can promote bone loss. Always opt for caffeine-free soft drinks, which won't act as a diuretic or cause your blood sugar levels to sky rocket.

111. TOFU TWO?
For variation in your diet and to reduce your intake of saturated fat, occasionally use tofu in recipes instead of meat. Tofu is made from soya beans so it's a great protein source, especially for vegetarians and vegans. It also absorbs flavours well, so marinate it before cooking or serve it with a tasty sauce.

112. SOY SIMPLE
Add a dash of flavour to soups, stir-fries and casseroles with soy sauce, or use it as a marinade. Although soy sauce is high in salt, only a very small amount is needed for intense flavour, so no other salt is required. Choose light or reduced-salt varieties and, as soy sauce frequently contains wheat, look for wheat-free versions if you suffer from an intolerance or coeliac disease.

113. MARINADE MASTERCLASS
Instead of using creamy, high-fat sauces, marinate chopped meat, chicken, fish or tofu (with a small amount of cornflour to help it stick better) in a resealable plastic bag. A little jiggle of the bag will distribute the marinade, leaving you with no washing up.

114. CREAMY TARRAGON CHICKEN
This tasty, low-fat dish is quick and easy to prepare. Fry two chicken fillets, chopped into small chunks, with garlic and mushrooms. Add 500ml (18fl oz) reduced-fat crème fraiche and simmer until the chicken is cooked. Add some tarragon and freshly ground black pepper, then serve with cooked rice or pasta and your vegetables of choice. Serves two.

115. YOU SAY POTATO . . .
For a low GI alternative to ordinary potatoes, try sweet potatoes. Bake, boil or roast them and add them to soups as a thickener. Throw some in with ordinary potatoes when boiling them, then combine for a tasty alternative to plain mash.

116. SPICY, HEALTHY FRIES
Cut two baking or sweet potatoes into wedges, leaving the skin on. Toss in some olive oil and sprinkle liberally with paprika. Bake at 180°C (350°F/Gas Mark 4) for 25 minutes, turning halfway through.

117. SUPER SQUASH
Pumpkin and butternut squash are packed with antioxidant vitamins A, C and E. Wash and roast pumpkin seeds for a healthy snack. Roast chopped pumpkin or butternut squash with other vegetables as a side dish, or add them to soups as a thickener.

118. POLENTA
Polenta, also known as cornmeal, is gluten and wheat free. Buy instant polenta and serve it with tomato dishes as you would pasta or rice, or use it as a coating in recipes that call for flour. Polenta is low in fat and calories, but watch out for ingredients that are added to flavour it, such as parmesan or butter.

119. TASTY TURKEY BURGER
For a low-fat alternative to beef burgers, mix 450g (1lb) minced turkey, half a red pepper and half a red onion, both finely chopped, 2 Tbsp chopped fresh parsley, one beaten egg and 40g (1½oz) breadcrumbs. Divide the mixture into four burgers and grill for 10–12 minutes, or until they are cooked through.

120. FRUITS OF LABOUR

Nearly all fresh fruits are low GI, except for those that are particularly high in sugar and low in fibre (e.g. melons). These fruits are digested quickly, resulting in a high GI rating. Ripe bananas are quite high in sugar but are also high in fibre, which lowers their GI value. Green bananas are slightly lower GI, as they aren't as high in sugar.

121. KEEP YOUR STRENGTH UP

Illness is often coupled with a loss or reduction of appetite. Try to eat little and often, concentrating on nutritious comfort foods like soup, smoothies, mashed potatoes and puréed vegetables.

122. FROZEN FANCY

Swap ice cream for frozen yoghurt, which is low in fat. If you can't find frozen yoghurt in your supermarket, add some mixed berries to regular yoghurt and freeze. Allow the mixture to defrost slightly before you eat it.

123. PIZZA THE ACTION

Make a frozen Margherita pizza healthier by adding chopped peppers, mushrooms and onions. Avoid meat toppings, especially pepperoni, or add your own meat in the form of lean or Parma ham. Always choose a thin base rather than stuffed or thick bases.

124. SAVING UP

Healthy eating doesn't mean spending more money. You might even save money if you shop wisely. Cut convenience foods and buy fresh vegetables, not pre-prepared ones. Choose supermarket own brands and buy in bulk. By shopping later in the evening, you can usually pick up bargains on bread, vegetables and meat.

NUTRITION AND HEALTH

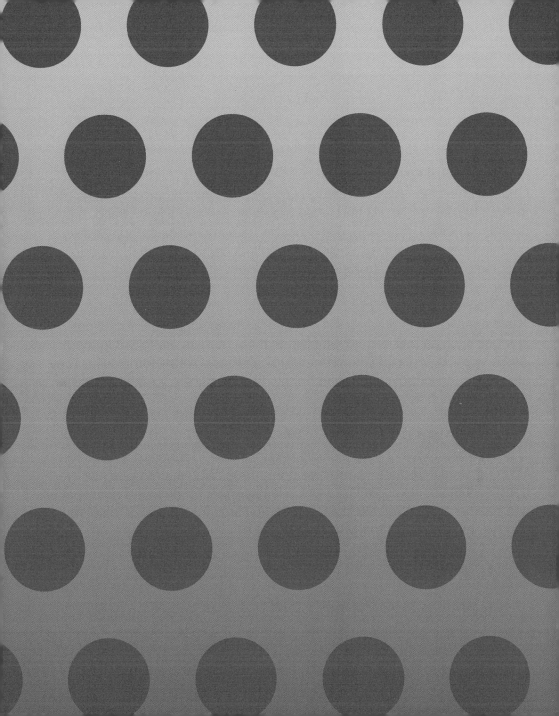

125. BE UNREFINED

Choose unrefined, complex carbohydrates over refined carbohydrates. So instead of cakes, biscuits and white bread, go for wholegrain bread, breakfast cereals, potatoes, pulses, rice and pasta. These complex carbohydrates contain all or most of their original nutrients and should form the bulk of your diet.

126. SWEETEN UP

There are two types of sugars in our diet. Intrinsic sugars are found naturally in foods such as fruit and vegetables. Extrinsic sugars are found in foods to which sugar is added during processing, such as cakes and biscuits. They are also found in table sugar and honey. Try to reduce your intake of extrinsic sugars as much as possible.

127. THE F WORD

There are two types of fibre: soluble and insoluble. Both are good for you. Sources of each include vegetables and pulses. Wheat, corn and rice are good sources of insoluble fibre, which is important for avoiding constipation and haemorrhoids. Soluble fibre is found in citrus fruits, apples, oats, barley and rye, and may help to lower cholesterol.

128. STAY REGULAR

You probably don't get enough fibre in your diet – most of us don't (see tip 127). As well as protecting against various ailments, fibre fills you up for longer. An intake of 20–24g (¾–1oz) each day is optimum. Have it with a glass of water, which bulks up the fibre so that it passes through your body more easily.

129. FAT'S NOT ALL BAD

Despite the bad rap it gets, you do need some fat in your diet. Fat provides energy, protects your organs and helps with the absorption of the fat-soluble vitamins A, D, E and K. Polyunsaturated fats supply essential fatty acids (see tip 131), which can't be made in the body and so must be obtained from your diet.

130. CALORIE COUNT

The excess calories that you eat are stored as fat, so to lose weight or maintain a healthy weight, your calories consumed should equal calories burned (see tips 421 and 427). Calorie requirements differ across age groups and genders, but on average women require 1,900–2,000 calories, and men 2,500 calories, each day. Fat provides 7 calories per gram; protein and carbohydrates provide 4 calories each per gram; and alcohol provides 9 calories per gram.

131. SOMETHING FISHY
More commonly known as Omega 6 and Omega 3 fatty acids, essential fatty acids keep your heart healthy, may protect against some cancers and relieve arthritis. They may also boost brain power and improve symptoms of attention deficit hyperactivity disorder (ADHD) in children, so eat plenty. The following foods are rich in Omega 6 and Omega 3 fatty acids:

- mackerel
- herring
- salmon
- fresh tuna
- walnuts
- Brazil nuts
- sunflower oil

132. BEWARE OF TRANS FATS
Trans fats, also known as hydrogenated fats, act like saturated (bad) fats in the body, so avoid them! Studies have shown that trans fats can raise levels of bad (LDL) cholesterol and reduce levels of good (HDL) cholesterol. They are mainly found in fast foods, margarines and baked goods.

133. SOURCES OF SATURATED FATS
Saturated fats increase levels of bad (LDL) cholesterol, at the same time increasing your risk of heart disease. Limit your intake of the following foods, which contain saturated fats in abundance:

- butter
- double cream
- bacon
- full-fat cheese
- shortcrust pastry
- potato crisps

134. MAKING THE MOST OF MONO

Replacing saturated and trans fats in your diet with monounsaturates (good fats) could lower your levels of bad (LDL) cholesterol and may even slightly increase levels of good (HDL) cholesterol. Look for Mediterranean recipes: the Mediterranean diet is linked with reduced incidences of heart disease and some cancers. The following foods are rich sources of monounsaturates:

- olive oil
- rapeseed oil
- sesame oil
- almonds
- Brazil nuts
- hummus
- avocado
- mackerel

135. BUILDING BLOCKS OF LIFE

Protein is required for growth, development, maintenance and repair of all body cells and tissues. The following foods are good protein sources:

Animal sources:

- meat
- poultry
- fish
- eggs
- cheese
- milk
- yoghurt

Vegetable sources:

- soya beans
- peanuts
- quinoa
- lentils
- kidney beans
- tofu
- wholemeal bread

136. UP THE ANTI!

An antioxidant is a compound that prevents damage or breakdown of body cells and tissues by oxidation and free radicals. Free radicals have been linked to ageing and diseases such as cancer and heart disease. Many vitamins act as antioxidants, which is why it's so important to eat plenty of fruit and vegetables.

137. EASY AS ABC

You can't see them because they're present in tiny amounts in foods – but without vitamins, you wouldn't survive. As well as A, B and C, there's also D, E and K. And there's more – there are at least 6 vitamins in the B group alone! Check out the tips on these two pages for the lowdown on what they all do and the best food sources.

138. VITAMIN A – RETINOL

Retinol is essential for healthy vision, skin and growth. A deficiency can lead to poor vision and eventually blindness. Retinol is found in animal sources such as milk, butter, cheese, eggs and oily fish. (Vegans needn't worry; they get enough vitamin A in their diets in the form of beta carotene.) Excessive intakes can be toxic, and pregnant women are advised not to take high-dose vitamin A supplements.

139. VITAMIN A – BETA CAROTENE

Beta carotene is an important antioxidant as it is believed to reduce the risk of cancer and heart disease, and also slows down the ageing process. Good sources include carrots, sweet potatoes, red peppers, green vegetables and tomatoes. The more colourful the food on your plate, the better!

140. B IS FOR BOOST
Vitamins B1, B2, B3, B6, B12 and folate work together in the body to aid growth and repair of the nervous system, digestion and the release of energy from food. In addition, they all have individual functions and can be found in foods such as fortified breakfast cereals, yeast extract, sunflower seeds, fish and eggs.

141. FANTASTIC FOLATE
Folate deserves a mention all of its own because it is so important in preventing birth defects. Women of child-bearing age should take a folate supplement of 400mg each day. Get it in your diet from spinach and other green vegetables.

142. C FOR CITRUS
Another antioxidant, vitamin C boosts immunity and builds and maintains healthy skin. It also helps in the healing of fractures and wounds. You'll find vitamin C in abundance in most fruits and vegetables, especially kiwi fruits, blackcurrants, oranges, peppers and broccoli.

143. VITAMIN D
Vitamin D helps with the absorption of calcium and so is responsible for the formation of strong, healthy bones and teeth. Too much vitamin D can be harmful, so high-dose supplements are not advisable. Vitamin D is made by the action of sunlight on your skin, and it is found in small amounts in oily fish, dairy products and fortified margarines.

144. VITAMIN E

A very powerful antioxidant, vitamin E protects against the build-up of plaque in the arteries, therefore helping to prevent heart disease. It also helps in the fight against ageing and may reduce the risk of cancer. A regular intake of polyunsaturated fats like sunflower oil and seeds, cod liver oil, rapeseed oil and pine nuts will ensure you're getting enough vitamin E.

145. VITAMIN K

Vitamin K is necessary for the normal clotting of blood. It can be made in the body, so deficiency is rare, but it can also be obtained in your diet from green, leafy vegetables, egg yolks, fish and yoghurt.

146. ELEMENTARY, MY DEAR

The minerals that you need from your diet in the greatest quantities include iron, calcium, magnesium, potassium, sodium, phosphorus and zinc. Other minerals are needed in smaller quantities but are just as important, and include selenium, copper, iodine and fluoride. The tips on these two pages give you an overview of essential minerals.

147. IRON IT OUT

The best sources of iron include red meat, seaweed, lentils, sesame and pumpkin seeds, green, leafy vegetables and fortified breakfast cereals. Iron is an essential component of haemoglobin, which carries oxygen round the body, so it's extremely important that you are getting enough in your diet.

148. PARTNERS IN IRON

Vitamin C aids iron absorption, so always try to pair vitamin C-packed foods and iron-rich foods. For example, have a glass of orange juice with your breakfast cereal, eat plenty of vegetables with your meat or snack on an orange after your meals.

149. NO BONES ABOUT IT

Calcium is the mineral that is needed in the greatest quantities. It keeps your bones and teeth strong, and ensures proper functioning of muscles and nerves. The main sources of calcium in the diet are dairy products, leafy green vegetables, beans and pulses, nuts and seeds, and even fortified foods such as breakfast cereals and calcium-fortified orange juice. Don't forget that Vitamin D helps with the absorption of calcium (see tip 143).

150. Z IS FOR ZINC

Zinc is essential for normal growth and development, a healthy reproductive system and fertility. It keeps your skin healthy, aids the healing of wounds and also has antioxidant properties. Get your zinc from meat, dairy products, wholegrain cereals, pulses, nuts and seeds.

151. SUPER SELENIUM

Selenium is an antioxidant and has been shown to protect against heart disease, cancers and premature ageing. It may also help to relieve pain in arthritis sufferers. Selenium works in conjunction with vitamin E (see tip 144) to ensure fertility and healthy growth, skin and hair. Both vitamin E and selenium are found in Brazil nuts and sunflower seeds. Selenium is also found in fish such as tuna, which can be eaten with sweet potatoes to provide vitamin E.

152. UNDER PRESSURE WITH POTASSIUM

Potassium regulates the heartbeat, nerves and blood pressure, and a severe deficiency can cause heart problems. Together, potassium and sodium regulate body fluids and can lower high blood pressure. Low-sodium, potassium-rich foods include bananas, nuts, pulses, potatoes and dried fruits.

153. BEWARE THE FIZZ

Diet can prevent or promote tooth decay. Avoid a high intake of foods like sweets and fizzy drinks, as these encourage bacteria to produce acid that dissolves tooth enamel, causing cavities. Protect teeth against erosion by finishing a meal with an alkaline food such as a glass of milk or a matchbox-sized piece of cheese.

154. FLUORIDE TOOTHPASTE

Fluoride is necessary for healthy bones and teeth. There is little risk of deficiency, as it is often added to water supplies, but a daily brushing with fluoridated toothpaste helps.

155. PHYTING FIT

Fruit and vegetables are good for you. They contain phytonutrients, which have antioxidant properties. Eat a wide variety of these foods to reduce your risk of cancer, heart disease and infection, and to step up immunity.

156. BOTTOMS UP!

Moderate intakes of alcohol, in particular red wine, are believed to reduce the risks of heart disease, cancer and Alzheimer's disease. Red wine also increases the levels of good (HDL) cholesterol in the body and decreases the levels of bad (LDL) cholesterol. It may also boost longevity, so drink up (in moderation!) for a longer, healthier life.

157. DON'T OVERDO IT

Despite its potential health benefits, alcohol is a drug with the power to become addictive. One or two units each day are optimum for obtaining the benefits it has to offer. Consistently drinking four or more units a day will negate these benefits and may actually increase health risks associated with high intakes of alcohol. Try to limit your daily intake to no more than one or two units.

158. KNOW YOUR LIMITS

It's better to spread your alcohol intake over the week, rather than binge drinking on one or two occasions. Know your limits and don't drink on an empty stomach, as the alcohol will take effect much faster. Men should drink no more than 21 units each week, and women should drink no more than 14 units.

159. KEEP THE PRESSURE DOWN

High blood pressure (hypertension) can increase your risk of heart disease and stroke. Your doctor will advise you if you need medication for your blood pressure, but diet can also help. Try to avoid foods with a high salt content (see tip 34).

160. IS YOUR NUMBER UP?

Get your cholesterol checked at least twice a year, especially if you have a family history of high cholesterol or heart disease. You do need some cholesterol in your diet, but if your levels are too high, cut down on red meat and limit eggs to no more than four each week.

161. AT THE WATERING HOLE

Your body is made up of approximately 70 per cent water, so it's important to keep this level topped up. Since you lose around 2 litres (3½ pints) of water each day just by breathing, perspiring and going to the toilet, you need to try to drink at least an equivalent amount every day to replace the water that is lost. Be aware that diuretics encourage the loss of water and overwork your kidneys. Tea, coffee and some soft drinks like cola contain caffeine, which is a common diuretic; alcohol is an even stronger diuretic.

162. MELLOW YELLOW

Check the colour of your urine for a guide to how dehydrated you are. First thing in the morning, you will be more dehydrated, so your urine will be a strong yellow colour. The rest of the time you should be aiming for a pale yellow colour.

163. WATER WORKS

Drink still rather than sparkling water. It's much easier to digest than its fizzy counterpart, which can cause bloating and may even encourage cellulite. If you really don't like the taste of plain water, add some fresh lemon or lime juice rather than a sugar-filled cordial. Water at room temperature is easier to drink than chilled water.

164. ECO-FRIENDLY

Bottled water is relatively inexpensive, but the cost of buying it every day adds up over the course of a year. If your tap water isn't up to scratch, filter it at home to make it taste better and balance the mineral content. This is also much more environmentally friendly than buying bottled water.

165. PILLS AND POTIONS

Provided you aren't pregnant and eat a healthy, balanced diet, you shouldn't have to boost your nutrient intakes with supplements. However, there's no harm in taking a multivitamin and mineral supplement every three or four days. (There's really no need to take supplements every day.) If you are prescribed supplements by your doctor, take them as directed. Otherwise, follow these tips for buying and taking them:

- Don't take daily doses of vitamins and minerals that exceed the safe upper limits. (Check your department of health's website for your country's prescribed amounts.)
- Tell your doctor about your supplements if you are seeing him or her about a health concern.
- Avoid supplements for weight control or weight loss (see tip 312).
- Don't just take something because it's working for your friend – do some research.
- Be aware of potential adverse reactions.

166. GI JANE

GI stands for glycaemic index. This is a method of numbering carbohydrate foods to tell you if a particular food will make your blood sugar levels rise very quickly, moderately or very slowly. Low GI foods release energy more slowly than high GI foods. Here are some of the benefits of eating the GI way:

- feel fuller for longer
- boost energy levels
- re-fuel your carbohydrate stores after exercise
- reduce cravings
- control blood sugar and insulin levels
- manage diabetes
- lose weight

167. TOP TEN LOW GI FOODS

- sweet potatoes
- beans
- rye bread
- peppers
- brown basmati rice
- strawberries
- dark chocolate
- broccoli
- pasta
- lentils

168. GLUTEN-FREE GREEN LIGHT

If you suffer from coeliac disease, you'll know how important it is to avoid gluten in your diet. Check labels and concentrate on what you can eat, rather than what you can't eat. Base your diet around lean protein foods, fruit and vegetables, rice, potatoes, quinoa and low-fat dairy products.

169. BREAST IS BEST

Breastfeeding helps you form a bond with your baby immediately and is the best form of nutrition. It establishes the baby's immune system, reduces the risk of infection early in life and may prevent obesity later in life. Breastfeeding your baby even for a short time will benefit his or her health. It will also help you lose any weight gained during pregnancy.

170. DIABETES AND DIET

If diabetes runs in your family, you can take steps to avoid developing it later in life. Maintaining a healthy weight, cutting down on your sugar intake and following a GI diet will all help reduce the risk of diabetes.

171. IRRITATING IBS

Bloating, cramps, diarrhoea, constipation – if you suffer from some or all of these on a regular basis, you may have irritable bowel syndrome (IBS). Stress and diet are common triggers. To identify problematic foods, keep a food diary as well as a record of symptoms. You'll be able to establish patterns and will know what foods to avoid.

172. DIABETIC DILEMMA

Don't be tempted by specialist 'diabetic' foods such as jams and chocolates. These products have the same effect on blood sugar as the regular products and have similar calorie values. Instead, choose high-fruit jams and, if you must have chocolate, have a small amount of dark chocolate, which has less sugar.

173. NOT UP TO IT

Loss of appetite often follows illness, shock or periods of anxiety and is common in the elderly and young children. To tempt a poor appetite, graze on small amounts of tasty, attractive foods frequently. Avoid low-nutrient 'junk' foods and don't indulge in large drinks before meals.

174. GOING ROUND IN CIRCLES

Poor circulation is signalled by pale hands and feet, digestive problems and a feeling of weakness. Exercise and including garlic, ginger and oily fish in your diet will improve circulation. Supplements containing vitamin E, fish oils and linseed oil will also help.

175. FEED A COLD

Although vitamin C is associated with preventing colds, this has never been scientifically proven. Increasing your vitamin C intake through supplementation when you feel a cold coming on should reduce its severity and duration, however. Garlic, ginger and chilli also relieve symptoms. Even though you may not feel like it, make sure you drink plenty of fluids while you are ill to maintain hydration.

176. CRANBERRY POWER

Cystitis is a painful urinary tract infection. The sufferer feels the need to urinate frequently, but can only pass a few drops at a time and experiences a burning sensation when passing urine. Drink reduced-sugar cranberry juice to prevent and relieve symptoms. It is also important to drink plenty of water to dilute the urine and make it easier to pass.

177. ECZEMA AND DIET

Some foods, such as milk, cheese, eggs, citrus fruits, food additives and tomatoes, are believed to make eczema worse. Try excluding them from your diet for a while to see if your symptoms improve. Evening primrose oil and fish oil supplements can also minimize symptoms of eczema and psoriasis.

178. FIGHTING FATIGUE

Fatigue, or feeling tired all the time, can have many causes, including an underlying health condition, depression, menopause or diet. Try cutting down on caffeine, alcohol and sugar, and eating small, regular meals. If that doesn't help, speak to your doctor if you are experiencing abnormal levels of tiredness.

179. WINDY DAYS

Excess wind, or flatulence, can be uncomfortable and embarrassing. Diet is usually the cause and is also the key to minimizing it. Here are some tips:

- Chop up your food into small pieces and chew it slowly.
- Eat with your mouth closed to avoid swallowing excess air.
- Purée foods like vegetables to break down the fibre.
- Thoroughly cook foods like beans and pulses.
- Drink peppermint or ginger tea after meals to aid digestion.
- Take a probiotic supplement – it aids digestion.

180. WATERED DOWN

Extra fluid in the body manifests itself as puffy ankles and bloated tummy, face and hands. Women often suffer from fluid retention round the time of menstruation or during menopause. To prevent it, drink plenty of water and follow a low-salt diet (see tip 34).

181. BREATHE EASY

Bad breath is another embarrassing condition but it can easily be treated by a change in diet and improved oral hygiene.

- Avoid eating strong-tasting foods like garlic and curries.
- Chew parsley or mints after eating to neutralize odours.
- Floss regularly and use a tongue scraper when cleaning your teeth, as nasty-smelling bacteria can attach themselves to your tongue.
- Drink lots of water and, if the condition persists, speak to your dentist for advice.

182. SUGAR EXTREMES

Poor dietary habits or long periods of exercise without eating can cause blood sugar levels to drop dangerously low (aka hypoglycaemia). This can cause dizziness, weakness, sweating, palpitations and nausea. If you experience any of these symptoms, control them by following a GI diet (see tip 166) and eat small amounts, often.

183. THAT TIME AGAIN

If heavy periods are a problem for you, iron supplementation may be necessary – your doctor will be able to advise. Absence of periods can be a sign of stress, excessive exercising or undereating. To prevent water retention when your period is due, avoid high salt intakes and drink plenty of water. Evening primrose oil supplements are thought to relieve premenstrual syndrome (PMS).

184. CREAKY BONES

If you suffer from arthritis, eliminate foods from the nightshade family from your diet for a few days. Avoiding potatoes, aubergines, tomatoes, courgettes and peppers can dramatically reduce pain. Citrus fruits are thought to exacerbate soreness owing to their acidity, so cut down on these, too. Glucosamine and fish oil supplements may relieve stiffness and inflammation.

185. DOZING OFF

Insomnia can be very frustrating and distressing for a sufferer and anyone who shares his or her bed. It is usually related to stress or anxiety, so relaxation techniques may help, as will regular exercise. Diet can also play a part – insomniacs should avoid coffee, tea, cola, alcohol, red meat and cheese in the evenings.

186. REMEMBER IT WELL

Eating a healthy, balanced diet throughout your life will keep your memory in top condition. Eating fish and taking fish oil supplements are associated with a decreased risk of developing Alzheimer's disease, and Gingko biloba supplements are believed to improve memory and boost brain function.

187. COOL DOWN YOUR DIET

Mouth ulcers are related to stress and diet. If you suffer from them, eat neutral foods like natural yoghurt. Avoid spicy and acidic foods like vinegar, tomatoes, salad dressings, curries and citrus fruits.

188. IN THE FAMILY WAY

If you're planning to conceive, here's what you can do to help things along:
- Lose weight – obesity can cause infertility by hampering ovulation, so losing weight through healthy eating should increase your chances of conception.
- Take folic acid – all women of child-bearing age should take a folic acid supplement of 400mg each day to prevent neural tube defects like spina bifida in their unborn child.
- Boost zinc intake – male fertility can be improved with zinc-rich foods such as Brazil nuts, meat and wholegrains.
- Cut down on alcohol, caffeine and smoking.

189. EATING FOR TWO

Being pregnant doesn't mean that you have to eat for two – energy requirements only increase in the last trimester by 200 calories each day. Being overweight during pregnancy carries health risks for both mother and baby, so you should continue to eat a balanced diet and take regular exercise. Ask your doctor or midwife for more detailed advice.

190. NURSING NEEDS

Breastfeeding uses at least 500 calories a day, so a bigger appetite is to be expected and should be satisfied with nutritious foods. Your body's requirements for protein, calcium, folate and vitamins C and A increase significantly during this time. Drink plenty of water and don't ignore thirst. Avoid drinking excessive amounts of tea, coffee and alcohol, as these are all excreted in your breast milk.

191. BRUISED AND BATTERED

Wound healing can be aided by an adequate intake of vitamins C and E (see tips 142 and 144). Alternatively, burst open a vitamin E capsule and massage the oil directly onto your wound. Honey is also an excellent antiseptic and can be applied to inflamed areas.

192. KIDDING AROUND

Young children, from the time of weaning to the age of five, need lots of calories and nutrients owing to their high activity levels and rapid growth. Include a wide variety of foods in your children's diets so that healthy habits are established early.

193. MANAGING MENOPAUSE

Menopausal symptoms vary in their type and severity. Ensure you have an adequate calcium intake and try vitamin E supplements to control hot flushes. Avoid fluid retention through a low-sodium diet supplemented with plenty of water.

194. SCREEN SAVER

Even if you seem to be in perfect health, it's important to get checked out regularly, especially after your 50th birthday. Ask your doctor about the screening tests that are available to you. Mammograms, cervical smears, screening for cancers, cholesterol checks and diabetes tests, to name but a few, can all save lives.

WEIGHT LOSS

195. DIET PERFECTION

Diet is defined as 'what you usually eat', not 'what you eat when you want to lose weight'. The 'diet' that's best for you is the one that you can maintain for life.

196. STRIKING A BALANCE

A balanced diet should consist of a variety of foods: lots of fruit, vegetables and starchy foods such as wholemeal bread and wholegrain cereals; some lean protein foods like meat, fish and lentils; and some low-fat dairy foods. You should also leave room for the odd treat.

197. JOIN THE CLUB

For help and motivation with your weight loss, why not join a diet club? If you can't face going to weekly public meetings, have a look at weight-loss programmes on the Internet. They offer online forums so you can get in touch with your peers and still have support, all from the comfort of your own home.

198. BMI BASICS

BMI (body mass index) compares your height to your weight and is a simple way of assessing whether you need to lose weight. To calculate your BMI, take your height in metres and multiply it by itself. Then divide your weight in kilograms by this figure.

199. CATEGORICAL

Here's what your BMI means, according to the World Health Organisation (WHO):

- Less than 18.5 = underweight
- 18.5–24.9 = normal weight
- 25– 29.9 = overweight
- over 30 = obese

The higher your BMI is over 30, the greater the risks to your health – so losing weight is not just about enhancing your physical appearance, it's about improving your overall health and well-being.

200. APPLES AND PEARS

These are the two basic body shapes. Apple-shaped people tend to carry a lot of weight around their middles, which increases their risk of heart disease and diabetes. Pear-shaped people carry weight on their hips but have fewer health complaints than apple shapes, even if they are overweight.

201. WAIST AWAY

Divide your waist measurement (at its narrowest point) by your hip measurement (at its widest point) to calculate your waist to hip ratio. Ratios above 0.80 for women, and 0.95 for men, may increase your risk of health complications and diseases. Weight loss will help reduce these health risks.

202. BODY FAT

Some weighing scales also measure body fat. While these calculations are not entirely accurate, they can give you a good idea of your body-fat percentage and help you see how eating healthily and exercising can reduce it. The average healthy adult's body fat is 15–18 per cent for men and 22–25 per cent for women.

203. BLAME GAME

Don't blame your metabolism for your weight. Metabolism is the amount of calories you burn at rest, or the amount of energy your body uses to function. Larger people actually have a faster metabolism than thinner people, and contrary to popular belief there is no magic method for speeding up metabolism. Exercising and eating frequent, small meals boost metabolism, but eating too few calories has the opposite effect.

204. STOCKTAKING

Examine the contents of your kitchen cupboards and get rid of anything that doesn't fit in with a healthy way of eating. Take tempting biscuits, crisps, cakes and sweets to work or to a neighbour, then restock with a trolley-full of healthy foods.

205. GOOD, BAD, UGLY

There are no such things as good and bad foods. Just because you've cleared your kitchen cupboards of unhealthy foods doesn't mean you can never have them again. It's all about finding a balance and treating yourself in moderation.

206. THE D WORD

Never say things like: 'I'm on a diet' or 'When I come off my diet'. Diet is not a train going up and down a track; it's a one-way trip to a healthy lifestyle, which you will only achieve by making changes to your current lifestyle without looking back.

207. BACK UP PLAN

Tell a close friend that you want to lose weight and are embarking on a healthy regime to do so. When you feel your resolve weakening, phone your friend for support and reassurance that you can do this. By the time you get off the phone, your craving will have passed!

208. OVERCOME OBSESSION

Don't spend your day obsessing about calories. Choose a weight-loss plan that suits you and spend a week or so getting your head around it and familiarizing yourself with the portions. Once you're better educated, it will become part of your normal routine, and you won't have to check every single food label to find out how many calories you are eating. It doesn't matter if you go slightly under or slightly over some days.

209. PICKING AND CHOOSING

Okay, so you're not on a diet; you're making healthy lifestyle changes. But this doesn't mean you can't follow a plan to help you along. Choose a weight-loss plan that reflects your lifestyle. If you have little time for cooking, don't choose one with complicated recipes.

210. THINK OF THE CHILDREN

Make your children your biggest motivators. Being fit and healthy means you can keep up with them and have fun together. You'll also set good examples that will stay with your children for life.

211. TROLLEY DOLLY
Instead of shopping for bits and pieces of food every day, do a weekly or fortnightly shop in a large supermarket. It's much more economical, and if you go armed with a shopping list, you're less likely to buy unhealthy foods.

212. OUT OF SIGHT, OUT OF MIND
Don't buy foods that you know will tempt you. Avoid the confectionery aisle in the supermarket and steer clear of vending machines when you're out and about.

213. PERFECT PLATE
Fill half your plate with salad or vegetables, a quarter with lean protein and a quarter with carbohydrates. Keep sauces on the side so you can control the amount you eat.

214. POST IT
Write little notes for yourself and stick them round the house to help you stay on track. They could encourage you to go to your exercise class or remind you of some of the reasons why you want to lose weight.

215. GO THE WRITE WAY
It's easier to achieve something if you know why you're doing it. Write down why you want to succeed at weight loss – for example, for health reasons or because you want to be more active for your kids. Reminding yourself of these goals will keep you motivated.

216. GOALKEEPER

Do you know how much weight you want to lose or how quickly you can safely lose it? Set realistic, attainable goals and know what to expect, so you don't get frustrated and bail out before reaching your ideal weight. A healthy rate of weight loss is 1.3kg (3lb) to 2.2kg (5lb) in the first week and 0.4kg to 0.9kg (1–2lb) each week thereafter.

217. OBSTACLE COURSE

Now that you've set your goals, write down a list of obstacles that stand in your way. Decide how you can overcome them and make a note of that, too. For example, if you think eating takeaways has contributed to your weight gain, plan your meals for the week so you won't be tempted to order in.

218. PHOTO FIT

Stick a photo that will remind you why you want to lose weight on the fridge. It might be from last year's holidays when you realized that you didn't want to have to cover up on the beach next year. Use the photo to deter you from reaching into the fridge at every opportunity!

219. PLATEAU PROBLEMS

When you're trying to lose weight, it's common to hit a plateau, a stage when your weight simply stops moving. This can be very frustrating, but it could be a sign that your body is getting used to your new weight. Don't give up! Stick with the diet and exercise, and your weight loss will get back on track.

220. BREAKING THE CYCLE

If you're exercising and eating well but still aren't losing weight, try some of these tips:
- Drink more water.
- Increase the amount of exercise you're doing.
- Try some new recipes.

221. SEE-SAW

You will lose more weight some weeks than others. This doesn't mean you're doing something wrong; it's simply the nature of weight loss. For every week you remain the same weight, just remind yourself that the weight you've already lost is gone forever.

222. SCALE IT BACK
Don't be discouraged if your weight fluctuates day by day. Water content, constipation and even your meals can cause the daily changes reflected on the scale. To avoid confusion and disappointment, weigh yourself only once a week. Let how much healthier you feel and how your clothes are fitting be your 'scale.'

223. 80:20 RULE
Realistically, you won't stick to a diet plan all the time. For a greater chance of success, follow the 80:20 rule. Stick to good eating habits 80 per cent of the time, and for 20 per cent of the time, or roughly one day a week, indulge yourself without going overboard.

224. SMART SNACKING
Don't leave it to chance and end up having whatever is in the nearest vending machine – bring your own snacks when you're out and about. Choose foods that are packed in individual portion sizes to prevent overeating. A 125-g (4½-oz) pot of yoghurt, or biscuits and crackers that are wrapped in packets of twos or threes, are ideal.

225. BREAKFAST LIKE A KING
Research has shown that eating breakfast can help you control your weight. Filling up first thing will boost your energy levels and keep you from snacking unnecessarily later in the day. Have a bowl of wholegrain cereal or some wholegrain toast, a piece of fruit and a glass of juice to set you up for the day.

226. CEREAL KILLER
You might think that all cereals are healthy, but that's not necessarily true. Many are coated in sugar and have high levels of salt and not enough fibre. (Muesli, in particular, is guilty of this, so make sure you look for varieties with no added sugar.) Compare the labels on boxes and choose cereals that are high in fibre and low in sugar and salt.

227. WATER, WATER EVERYWHERE
When you're trying to lose weight, drink at least 1.5 litres (2¾ pints) of water every day. Keep a bottle of water on your desk at work and take one to the gym as well. You may even want to invest in a water purifier or a filter jug that fits in the fridge. These make your water taste better and balance the mineral content.

228. TAKE YOUR TIME
Spend plenty of time over your meals. The brain needs 20 minutes to register when your stomach is full, so take at least this much time over meals to prevent overeating. Take small bites, chew slowly and put down your cutlery between each mouthful.

229. STAND UP STRAIGHT

Good posture can make you look pounds lighter and boost your confidence. It also helps your breathing and maximizes energy levels. Stand sideways in front of a mirror and check out your posture. Now pull your shoulders back and see the instant difference. It's better for your back, too!

230. FILL UP, NOT OUT

Eating a diet rich in fibre will fill you up for longer and keep your calorie intake down. Swap chips for a baked potato, biscuits and cakes for fruit and fill up your plate with vegetables and salad at mealtimes to boost your fibre and overall nutrient intake. The more colourful the vegetables, the more nutritious they are!

231. ARE YOU REALLY HUNGRY?

If you feel like you need a snack, decide if you really are hungry before eating. Have a drink of water – your body often mistakes thirst for hunger. Don't eat out of boredom or because you're feeling emotional. Think about whether you really need this snack. More often than not, the answer will be no.

232. MEASURE UP

Although being overweight brings an increased risk to your health, it's important to be aware of where you deposit the extra weight. If you're female and your waist measurement is greater than 81cm (32in), or if you are male and your waist measurement is more than 94cm (37in), the greater the risk to your health and well-being.

233. THINK SMALL
Have five or six small meals throughout the day rather than the conventional two or three large meals. Eating this way stabilizes your blood sugar levels, making you feel fuller for longer so you won't be tempted to snack on foods that may jeopardize your weight loss.

234. IRREPLACEABLE
Avoid meal-replacement weight-loss plans. Although they may work well in the short-term, they do not teach you the importance of healthy eating and controlling portions for weight loss. They can also be expensive and may leave you at risk of nutritional deficiencies. Any weight you lose while following these plans is usually regained when you return to your normal diet.

235. BIT BY BIT
Small changes can alter your whole life. Plan three changes you can make right now – for instance, snack on fruit instead of biscuits or crisps; eat more vegetables; and swap white bread for wholegrain. When these have become everyday habits, move on to more small changes.

236. CALCULATE YOUR DRINKS
Give up the sugar in your coffee and switch to low-calorie drinks. It's amazing how many calories drinks can add to your daily intake. A glass of orange juice with breakfast contains 72 calories in 200ml (7fl oz); a coffee with sugar at breaktime, 20 calories; a can of coke in the afternoon, 129 calories; and a large glass of wine with dinner, approximately 200 calories.

237. BROADEN YOUR FOOD HORIZONS

If you've spied a strange-looking vegetable in your supermarket, find out what it is and how to cook it, then buy it. Keeping your food interesting will boost your enthusiasm for eating a healthy, balanced diet. After all, variety is the spice of life!

238. CHANGE YOUR ROUTINE

You might be a creature of habit, but even a small change in your daily routine will help you maintain a fresh outlook on life and prevent your lifestyle from becoming mundane. Try taking a new route to work, eat a pear instead of an apple or take the kids swimming instead of to the park.

239. OVEREATERS ANONYMOUS

Most people have triggers that will make them reach for the chocolate. Think about the reasons or the occasions that might cause you to overeat – for example, stressful moments at work or when you're watching television at night. When you've identified these triggers, you'll be able to prevent yourself from automatically eating at these times.

240. SATELLITE DISHES AND SAUCERS

The difference on your plate will translate to a difference on the scales. You might be eating healthy foods, but if you're eating too many of them, you won't lose weight. Be aware of how much you're eating and identify where you can cut down. Use a smaller plate so you'll be less likely to overfill it, and you'll save on calories.

241. SIZE MATTERS

Portion control is one of the keys to weight loss. Invest in a good set of kitchen scales and spend a week or two weighing foods until you get an idea of what portion sizes you should be eating. For example, weigh out 30g (1oz) of cereal. This is the recommended amount for a healthy breakfast – and you'll probably find that it's much less than what you've been eating.

242. ESTIMATING PORTIONS

Here's a rough estimate of the recommended portion sizes for some everyday foods. Again, do use the kitchen scales to get a more accurate idea.

- Seventy-five grams (2¾oz) of meat, poultry or fish is the same size as a deck of cards.
- Twenty-five grams (1oz) of cheese is the same size as a small box of matches.
- A serving of rice is half a teacup of uncooked rice.
- A medium potato is the size of a computer mouse.

243. SPICE IT UP

Make everyday foods like soups and baked potatoes more appealing by adding extra flavour with fresh herbs, spices or salsa. Give soup a kick with some dried chilli flakes, serve salsa with baked potatoes and add some fresh basil to a shop-bought tomato pasta sauce.

244. YOU'RE SWEET ENOUGH!

If you drink six cups of tea or coffee with sugar (16 calories per tsp) and whole milk (17 calories per 25ml/ 1fl oz) every day, it adds up to 200 calories. Bypass the sugar (use sweetener instead, if you like) and use skimmed or semi-skimmed milk, and you will automatically save yourself 150 calories!

245. NO ADDED SUGAR

Just because a food or drink says it has no added sugar or is sugar free doesn't mean it is calorie free. Products using these terms may contain sugar alcohols, a derivative of sugar that yield as many calories as table sugar (4 calories per gram).

246. MILKING IT

If you consume half a pint of milk each day (280ml/ 10fl oz), swapping to semi-skimmed will save you 56 calories and 5.6g (⅕oz) of fat each day. Over the course of a year, this could add up to a saving of 2.25kg (5lb) in body weight.

247. AVOID A STICKY SITUATION

Invest in some good-quality, non-stick saucepans and frying pans, which will eliminate the need for you to use oil or fat when you're cooking. When you're making foods like Bolognese sauce or chilli, dry fry the mince and drain off the extra fat before adding any sauce.

248. ONLY A FOOL!

Only you will know that you had that sneaky doughnut on the way home from work – but by eating in secret like this, you're only fooling yourself. The scales aren't going to lie to you, so be honest with yourself.

249. CLEAN PLATE CLUB

Cancel your membership to the clean plate club, because it's okay to leave food on your plate. You don't have to finish everything, so don't keep eating even when you're full. Keep leftovers for the next day, freeze them or give them to the dog – whatever it takes to keep you from eating them!

250. EAT IN PEACE

Reading, watching television or even talking during a meal all distract you from eating, so the likelihood is that you will overeat. Think about what you are eating and enjoy every mouthful. Eat slowly and stop eating when you are full.

251. THINK OUTSIDE THE LUNCHBOX

Bring your own lunch to work at least three days a week. You'll have total control over what you're eating and won't have to spend the morning worrying if there's something to suit your diet in nearby delis and cafés. If you only eat out once or twice a week, you'll also look forward to it more. Just make sure you stick to healthy choices or you'll undo all the good work you've achieved throughout the rest of the week.

252. MADE TO ORDER

Don't be afraid to ask for what you want, even at a fast food restaurant. Ask for salad instead of chips on the side; have either mayonnaise or butter on a sandwich, but not both; choose wholegrain bread rather than white; and ask for sauces and dressings to be served on the side.

253. NIP NIBBLING IN THE BUD

Nibbling and picking at food happens without you even realizing it, so the first step to stopping is to be aware of when you are doing it. Write down every single thing you eat, even when you only nibble on something, and you'll soon be able to identify why the weight is not falling off as fast as you'd like.

254. TICKING OVER

If you plan when you're going to eat throughout the day and vow to stick to those times, you're less likely to get distracted by food at other times and overeat. Plan to eat first thing in the morning, in mid-morning, at lunchtime, in mid-afternoon and at dinner- and supper-times.

255. DON'T CAVE IN TO CRAVINGS

Instead of giving in to a craving immediately, wait 20 minutes, and it will most likely pass. If the craving doesn't subside, you probably are hungry, so have something small to eat. If you're craving chocolate, have a couple of pieces rather than demolishing the whole bar.

256. DRIVEN TO DISTRACTION

When cravings strike, distract yourself with something else so you forget about food. Tackle the laundry or ironing, clean the bathroom, write a letter or phone a friend. The craving should pass in the meantime.

257. PURE INDULGENCE

Life would be very dull if you didn't have the odd treat, so allow yourself a bit of chocolate or a bag of crisps once or twice a week. By only treating yourself occasionally, you will look forward to it and appreciate it more.

258. LOW-CALORIE CHOCOLATE TREATS

- low-calorie hot chocolate drink
- 200-ml (7-fl oz) glass of chocolate milk
- low-fat chocolate mousse
- chocolate frozen yoghurt
- handful of chocolate raisins or peanuts

259. STRESSED OUT? GET ACTIVE!

Instead of comfort eating during stressful times, do some exercise. When you eat a high-fat or sugary food, chemicals called endorphins are released, making you feel good. Endorphins are also released during exercise, so choose to burn calories, lose weight and feel fantastic instead of consuming calories and possibly gaining weight!

260. PUMP SOME IRON

A pound of muscle burns up to nine times the calories that a pound of fat does, so turn some fat into muscle by including weight-bearing exercises in your workout. Weight training can also boost your metabolism, in turn helping you burn those calories.

261. DINING OUT

If you're going out for dinner, be prepared so you don't sabotage your weight-loss efforts. Many restaurants have their menus online, so get surfing and plan your meal to ensure you won't be tempted by fatty options when you get there.

262. STARVE OR STUFF?

Starving yourself before you dine out will only cause you to stuff yourself on high-fat and high-calorie foods when you reach the restaurant. Alcohol will also go to your head faster on an empty stomach. Have a healthy breakfast and lunch that day and a small snack before you leave for the restaurant so you won't eat too much.

263. FAT-FINDING MISSION

Watch out for fatty dishes on menus when you are eating out. 'Fried', 'crispy', 'au gratin', 'stuffed' and 'creamy' all denote extra calories and fat. Butter, cream, cheese, salami and other processed meats are high-fat ingredients, so avoid these, too.

264. DRESSING DOWN

Don't smother your salad in calorie-laden dressings. Keep dressing on the side of your plate and dip your fork into it before eating a forkful of salad. Better still, use lemon or lime juice for flavouring or a small amount of olive oil with balsamic vinegar.

265. NO APERITIF

Studies have shown that having a glass of alcohol before dinner will make you eat up to 200 calories more at dinner than you would have otherwise. Drinking with dinner may also cause you to eat more, so stick with water or, if you must have one, a small glass of wine.

266. CIAO, BELLA

If you're eating Italian food, steer clear of garlic bread, creamy sauces and risotto, which is cooked in lots of butter and cream. Avoid dishes with 'frito', 'alfredo', 'carbonara' or 'pepperoni' in their descriptions. Start with minestrone soup, salad or bruschetta. For your main course, opt for a tomato-based pasta dish or share a thin-crust pizza with vegetable toppings.

267. BON APPÉTIT

In a French restaurant, choose consommé or vegetable soup for your starter. For the main course, go with meat, fish or poultry without a heavy sauce, and served with salad or boiled potatoes. An omelette is also a good option – ask for vegetables to be added to yours. Paté, foie gras, escargot and French onion soup are all off limits, as are Dauphinoise or gratin potatoes. Wash down your healthy meal with a glass of antioxidant-rich red wine.

268. VIVA ESPAÑA

Choose gazpacho for a light, refreshing starter, though shellfish or a small portion of paella won't break the calorie bank. For the main course, a Spanish omelette with salad is an excellent choice, as are roast vegetables, beans and fish. Avoid sausage and cheese tapas, and watch the bread and olive oil portions – although a little of each is fine.

269. INDIAN SPICE

Avoid dishes made with cream or coconut, such as korma; a yoghurt- or tomato-based sauce is a better option. Tandoori dishes are a great choice because they are baked in an oven with spices but no sauce (or sauce comes on the side so you can control it). Dishes containing chick-peas and lentils also get the thumbs up. Order rice or naan for sides, but not both.

270. CHINESE WHISPERS

Avoid fried rice and crispy noodles, and dishes with 'crispy', 'battered', 'fried', 'dumpling' or 'satay' in their descriptions. Sweet-and-sour dishes are high in sugar and so are not GI friendly. Stir-fries made with hoi sin, black bean or ginger sauces and served with rice or noodles are good choices. Go easy with the soy sauce, though, as your dish is already likely to be high in salt.

271. TURNING JAPANESE

Japanese food is generally very healthy as it is low in fat and rich in vegetables and fish. Experiment with different types of sushi and choose rice and vegetable dishes such as cha han or ramen noodles. Avoid tempura dishes, which are battered and deep fried.

272. THAI BITES
Avoid dishes that contain peanuts or coconut milk. Stir-fried dishes with plenty of vegetables and lean chicken, beef or fish, served with ginger, garlic or chilli sauces, are good bets. Choose plain rice over rice that is fried or has been boiled in coconut milk.

273. FAST FOOD FEATURES
Don't assume that salads are a healthy option at fast food restaurants. Avoid the ones that contain crispy chicken or croutons and ask for the dressing to be served on the side. If you want a burger with your salad, choose a small one and hold the dressing and cheese. Have water or a diet soft drink instead of a calorie- and additive-laden milkshake.

274. SANDWICH SAVIOUR
Always request brown bread instead of white. Have a small amount of spread or mayonnaise but not both, or skip these and go for low-fat dressing or mustard instead. Choose lean protein fillings like turkey, ham, chicken, tuna, egg, cottage cheese or Swiss cheese. Pile on plenty of salad.

275. SALAD-BAR SABOTAGE
Bypass salads drenched in mayonnaise and dressing. Fill your plate with salad leaves, tomatoes, cucumber and other raw vegetables. Add protein in the form of cottage cheese, plain chicken, tuna or boiled eggs. Have some dressing on the side so you can control the amount you eat.

276. GET YOUR JUST DESSERTS

If you fancy something sweet after dinner, have some fruit salad, sorbet or a small amount of ice cream. Alternatively, share a dessert with someone else and go for a walk after dinner to burn off any excess calories.

277. CURIOSITY KILLED THE CAT

If you've made a decision not to have dessert or a glass of wine, don't torture yourself by asking for the dessert menu or wine list 'just for a quick look'. You'll more than likely end up giving into temptation.

278. SHARING IS CARING

If a certain starter or dessert on the menu has caught your eye, but you know that the portions at the restaurant are generous, ask someone dining with you if he or she would like to share. You only need to take a couple of bites, then you can leave your friend to finish off the rest.

279. PHONE A FRIEND

If you've been invited round to a friend's house for dinner, phone him or her in advance and mention that you're watching your weight. Offer to bring a dish, so you'll know what's in it, and ask your friend to give you smaller portions so no one will be offended if you don't eat everything during dinner.

280. MOVIE MUNCHIES

Going to the cinema can be a diet disaster, with all those supersize sweeties, sugary drinks and salty, buttered popcorn. Bring your own water and some air-popped popcorn or a small bar of chocolate, so you won't be tempted by the goodies on offer.

281. COFFEE CAPERS

If you can't curb your coffee habit, at least make it healthier. Ask for semi-skimmed or skimmed milk and skip the cream, marshmallows and sugar syrups. Have decaffeinated coffee occasionally and see if you can even notice the difference!

282. MAKE A COMEBACK

If you've strayed off your eating plan in a big way, you may feel out of control and unsure of how to get back on the healthy-eating wagon. Think about how you're feeling, and next time you're tempted to stray, ask yourself if that packet of biscuits is worth the feeling of guilt afterwards.

283. DON'T BE TOO HARD ON YOURSELF

Nobody's perfect, and you won't always be able to resist temptation. If this happens, put it behind you and start afresh. Don't ever starve yourself the day after a binge to make up for any extra calories you may have consumed.

284. TAKE RESPONSIBILITY

Ultimately, you are the only one who can make things happen for you. That means you are the one who has to make the plan; you are the one who needs to eat healthily and exercise each day; and you are the one who will have to overcome the hurdles to reach your goals. No one else can do this for you, so don't blame other factors for getting in the way.

285. WATCHING THE CLOCK
You've been working hard all morning, and suddenly it's lunchtime. You automatically unwrap your sandwich but realize you're not hungry. Don't eat it – yet! You don't have to eat just because it's lunchtime. Eat half the sandwich and save the rest for later, when you really are hungry.

286. RISE AND SHINE
Some people find that exercising in the morning regulates their appetite for the rest of the day. Try it and see if it applies to you. There's no right or wrong time to exercise, but if doing so first thing in the morning keeps your eating on track during the day, be an early bird!

287. BOOK CLUB
Read the biographies of people who inspire you. They don't have to have lost weight, but you can use their positive behaviour as inspiration to succeed with your own goals.

288. TAKE A NAP
If you've been burning the candle at both ends, your tiredness is probably making you feel stressed. This will cause your blood sugar to fluctuate, and you'll be more likely to want to snack on comfort foods. A short nap or some quiet time to yourself will reduce your stress levels and leave you feeling more energized.

289. CUT 100 CALORIES EACH DAY
It takes an excess of 3,500 calories to gain 450g (1lb), or 35,000 calories to put on 4.5kg (10lb) in a year. So, losing 4.5kg (10lb) can be as easy as eating 100 calories less each day for a year.

290. HOW TO CUT THOSE 100 CALORIES

- Cut out one slice of bread.
- Swap two full-fat yoghurts for two low-fat yoghurts.
- Exchange one sausage roll for two grilled sausages.
- Have two oranges instead of two glasses of orange juice.
- Choose a low-fat salad dressing instead of mayonnaise.

291. WOBBLY WEEKENDS

Routine tends to go out the window at weekends, but that doesn't mean that your good intentions have to go, too. If your weekend consists of takeaways, junk food and lounging in front of the television, ditch these habits and continue your healthy routine from Sunday to Sunday.

292. OPTICAL ILLUSION

Looking slim can simply be a case of styling yourself by choosing the right clothes for your figure. Here are some dos and don'ts:

- Wear heels to lengthen your legs and make your calves look slimmer.
- Knee-length dresses and skirts will elongate your legs, making you look taller and slimmer.
- Flatter curves with loose fabrics like chiffon.
- Avoid tapered trousers, as they emphasize the width of your hips.
- Don't wear tight-fitting clothes; they will cling in the wrong places.
- Stay away from horizontal stripes, which will make you look wider.
- Wear well-fitting underwear to avoid unsightly bumps and lumps.

293. COMPLIMENTARY CONFIDENCE

Compliments from other people about how good you look can be very motivating. Learn to accept compliments graciously. Instead of protesting, smile and say 'thank you'. Each time you receive a compliment, your confidence will soar.

294. HOW LOW CAN YOU GO

Eating too few calories will prevent you from losing weight. Women need at least 1,200 calories each day, and men at least 1,500 calories, to maintain basic bodily functions. Eat any less than this, and your body will go into starvation mode and your metabolism will slow down.

295. FAT'S LIFE

Fat should make up no more than 35 per cent of your total calorie intake. Buy foods with no more than 3–4g (⅛oz) of fat per 100g (3½oz). Remember, too, that 'fat free' doesn't mean 'calorie free', so check for high levels of sugar.

296. PACK IN THE PROTEIN

This isn't encouragement to go on a high-protein diet, but do make sure you have an adequate protein intake (see tip 135). Protein is harder for your body to break down than fat or carbohydrates, so you'll burn more calories by eating it. Protein also has a high satiety value, making you feel fuller for longer.

297. GET THE CONNECTION
It's not just food that influences your weight, but exercise, stress levels, sleeping patterns and hormones. Think about where you need to make changes in your life and you might just see a difference on the scales.

298. LONG HAUL
Even if you have a lot of weight to lose, split up your weight loss into small, manageable amounts. Mini-targets will help you stay motivated, so focus on losing 3kg (6lb 8oz) at a time and remember that a loss of 1kg (2lb 4oz) each week is a healthy and realistic rate of weight loss.

299. PENCIL THIN
Keep a food diary of everything you eat for a week or two. This should include all the food that you nibble and pick at throughout the day – like the chip you swiped from a colleague at lunchtime or the handful of grated cheese you munched while you were preparing dinner. You'll soon be able to identify where you're going wrong and the times that you're most likely to eat unconsciously.

300. NOTHING COMPARES
Don't compare your progress to that of someone else. Weight loss is different for everyone, and just because your friend is following the same diet and fitness plan as you, you won't necessarily progress at the same pace. Be your own competitor.

301. WHEN HUNGER CALLS
Don't deny yourself food when you're hungry; it's your body's way of telling you that you need fuel. Forgoing food until you're starving is also a bad idea, because you'll find it harder to control what you eat.

302. TRAVEL LIGHT
If you're on the move, plan ahead and take your food with you. The food that's available in airports, trains and service stations is notoriously limited, and often highly processed, so it won't do your fat and calorie intake any good. Always carry fruit, nuts, seeds and even sandwiches, so you'll never be caught short.

303. WAIST NOT, WANT NOT
If you're clearing up the dishes after a meal, put the scraps straight into the bin or the dog's dish. Don't be tempted to polish them off yourself – you won't realize you've done it and then you'll wonder why you're not losing weight.

304. TOP FIVE DIET MYTHS
It's time to realize once and for all that the following notions simply aren't true! See the tips on the opposite page to find out more about each myth.
- Celery has negative calories.
- Bread and pasta cause weight gain.
- Spicy foods burn fat faster.
- 'Fat free' means 'calorie free'.
- Eating late at night will cause weight gain.

305. NEGATIVE CALORIE NONSENSE

Contrary to popular belief, there is no such thing as a calorie- or fat-burning food. Although celery is very low in calories, you don't use up more calories chewing and digesting it than it contains. Unfortunately, this means it also won't cancel out the cake you ate earlier!

306. NO RED CARD FOR CARBS

Well, not unless you eat bread and pasta smothered in butter and creamy sauces all day long. It's the amount and type of carbohydrates that you eat that can affect your weight loss, so chose wholegrain breads and cereals, brown rice, potatoes and pasta. If you watch your portions, carbohydrates can still be included as part of your healthy-eating plan.

307. METABOLIC MYTHS

There's no truth in the old wives' tale that hot and spicy foods boost your metabolism, helping you burn fat faster. If spicy foods don't agree with you, rest assured that you're not missing anything. On the other hand, if you do want to spice things up, chuck in the chilli.

308. 'FAT-FREE' FALLACY

Many low-fat or fat-free foods are loaded with sugar, so always check their labels. Next time you're out shopping, compare the labels of low-fat biscuits with their ordinary equivalents and spot the differences.

309. FAST OR FEAST?

Calories are calories, no matter what time of day they are consumed. However, for a lot of people, late-night snacking usually means calorie-laden crisps or biscuits. If this sounds familiar, either eat healthier snacks or distract yourself so that you aren't tempted to nibble. Remember that no matter what time of day you eat crisps, they will have the same effect on your waistline.

310. BEAT POST-HOLIDAY BLOATING

Too much alcohol and lots of meals out can take their toll on your stomach and leave you feeling bloated and uncomfortable. Drink plenty of water and avoid processed foods for a week after returning from your holiday. Eat foods that are easy to digest, such as fish, mashed potatoes and puréed vegetables, and follow meals with a cup of peppermint tea.

311. CURB CRASH DIETING

If you suddenly crash down from 1,900 calories each day to 1,000 calories, your body will go into a state of shock. As a result, your metabolism will hold on to all available energy and fat stores, and you won't lose weight.

312. MONEY DOWN THE DRAIN

Pills proclaiming that they aid weight loss by blocking carbohydrates and fat are a complete waste of time. No peer-reviewed journals have published clinical studies showing long-term weight loss and management can be achieved by taking these pills. The only effect you're likely to experience is diarrhoea!

313. SNACKS WITH 10 CALORIES OR LESS

- sugar-free gum
- sugar-free jelly
- coffee or tea with skimmed milk
- water with slices of lemon or lime
- sugar-free flavoured sparkling water
- diet soft drinks
- herbal and fruit teas

314. SNACKS WITH 60–80 CALORIES OR LESS

- 20 grapes
- 300g (10½oz) air-popped popcorn spiced with cinnamon or paprika
- skinny latte or cappuccino (no added sugar)
- ten strawberries and 1 Tbsp Greek yoghurt
- two breadsticks and tomato salsa dip

315. SNACKS WITH 110–130 CALORIES OR LESS

- 20g (¾oz) mixed nuts
- 50g (1¾oz) dried fruit
- one slice wholegrain toast with 1 Tbsp peanut butter
- three celery sticks with 30g (1oz) reduced-fat hummus
- one pot low-fat yoghurt or fromage frais

316. FAST TRACK TO DANGER

Fasting for more than one day can be dangerous to your health and is certainly not the answer to permanent weight loss. Whether it's a 'water-only' fast used to detox, skipping meals or surviving on cabbage soup or grapefruit, the body goes into starvation mode, putting itself under stress. Regularly skipping meals can have a similar effect, so eat little and often.

317. YO-YO IS A NO-NO

Yo-yo dieting is where you chop and change from one (usually faddy) diet to another. This will throw your metabolism into chaos, and any weight lost on one diet is likely to be gained – with a bit extra – on the next one. Choose an eating plan that suits you and stick to it. This way, you're more likely to be successful.

318. FIGURE IT OUT

Though you can tone up and lose weight, you can't change your basic body shape, so you have to learn to be happy with it. Make the most of your figure by wearing well-fitting clothes and experiment with accessories to dress up any outfit.

319. BABY BUMP

If you're pregnant, you should not follow a weight-loss plan of any kind. Eat a healthy, balanced diet containing at least 2,000 calories each day. Dieting when you are breastfeeding is not recommended either, at least until the child is weaned and breast milk is not his or her only source of nutrition.

320. CHROMIUM CURE

If you find that you often crave carbohydrates or chocolate, try taking chromium supplements. Chromium regulates your blood sugar levels, so it might help curb the munchies. You can also get chromium in your diet from animal foods, fish and wholegrains, which partly explains why a low GI diet (see tip 166) helps prevent cravings.

321. MINTY FRESH

If you're feeling peckish, brush your teeth and rinse with mouthwash. You won't want to eat and, even if you do, the food won't taste nice because of the minty-fresh feeling in your mouth!

322. HYPOTHYROIDISM

Hypothyroidism occurs when the thyroid gland does not produce enough thyroid hormones. This tends to slow down the body's functions. Symptoms include tiredness, weight gain and sensitivity to the cold. It can be treated with medication, but weight loss may become difficult for sufferers. A low GI diet and exercise will slowly help with weight loss.

323. QUIET NIGHT OUT

Rather than always meeting friends at a bar, plan other activities that don't revolve around alcohol. Go to the cinema or theatre, or meet for a snack or a coffee in a nice café. You'll feel much better the next morning, and you can put the money saved towards a special treat for yourself.

324. SHIFTING THE BALANCE

Shift work can make it difficult to stick to a routine and cause problems with weight loss. Try to be prepared and take food with you instead of relying on high-fat vending machine snacks. Do some exercise in between shifts or during breaks.

325. NEVER SAY NEVER

Ban negative words like 'can't', 'won't' and 'never'. Associating food with negative words such as 'naughty', 'wicked' or 'forbidden' will only make you want them more. And instead of saying you're on a diet, say you're making 'healthy lifestyle changes'!

326. INCH BY INCH

If your weight loss has stalled, it may be that you are building muscle, which weighs more than fat. You can still drop clothes sizes even if the scales aren't moving. Measure your chest, waist and hips on a weekly basis as another indicator of success.

327. LOW-CARB LOWDOWN

Low-carbohydrate regimes can be useful for weight loss but are best for those with a lot of weight to lose. They are intended to be a long-term approach to weight loss and maintenance, so don't use a low-carbohydrate diet as a quick fix for losing weight. You'll only end up gaining it back, plus extra.

328. UNLOCK THE COMBINATION

Some diet plans are based around food combining – eating certain foods together, not eating certain foods together, only eating one type of food at each meal and so on. Sound crazy? It is. It doesn't matter what foods you combine. Weight loss is achieved by reducing overall calorie intake and eating a balanced diet. Forget faddy diets and concentrate on eating healthily.

329. SUPERMARKET SWEEP

Don't be tempted by special offers in the supermarket encouraging you to buy one item and get one free. These offers generally apply to unhealthy items like biscuits, pizzas and crisps. Shop later in the evening for reduced-price fruit, vegetables and bread.

330. GET REAL

Aspiring to look like your favourite celebrity is unrealistic and won't happen unless you are prepared to undergo major surgery! Be practical about the goals you set yourself so you know you will be able to achieve them.

331. IN FOR A PENNY, IN FOR A POUND

Start saving £1 for every 1kg (2lb 4oz) lost. When you've saved a decent amount, treat yourself with something nice – just not food! Try a new item of clothing or jewellery, a facial or a massage. You're worth it!

332. MEDICINE MAN

Although some medications can cause weight gain as a side effect, a calorie-controlled diet plan and exercise will help reduce this effect somewhat and still allow you to lose weight. Your rate of weight loss may be slightly slower, but don't be disheartened by this. You will get there.

333. SIGNS AND SIGNALS

Ways to measure progress without the scale:

- clothes feeling looser
- generally feeling healthier
- getting compliments
- increased activity levels

334. HAPPY HOLIDAYS

Going on holiday does not mean you have to forget all your good intentions. Aim for weight maintenance rather than loss, but keep an eye on your portions and stick to the same kinds of foods you usually eat. Keep active and have fun.

335. MAINTAINING WEIGHT

You've reached your target weight (well done!) and now you're wondering how you can maintain your weight. The trick is to continue eating the foods you've been eating but to eat more of them. Increase your calorie intake by 250 every week. If you're still losing weight, keep increasing the calories until you find the level that allows you to stay the same weight.

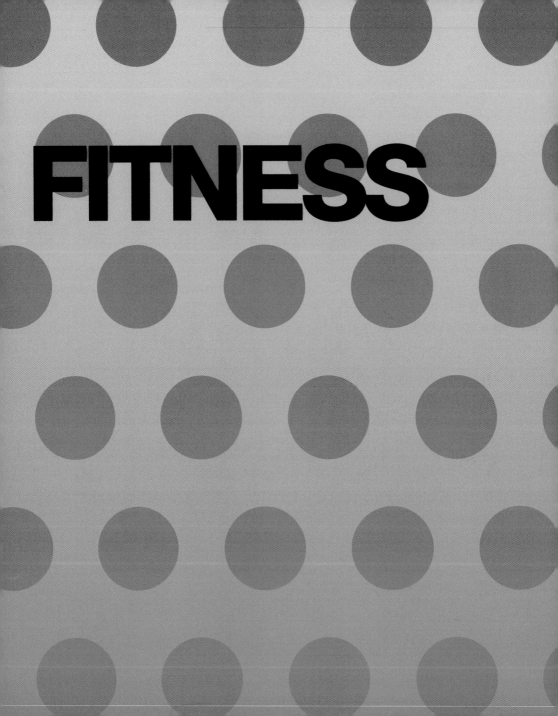

FITNESS

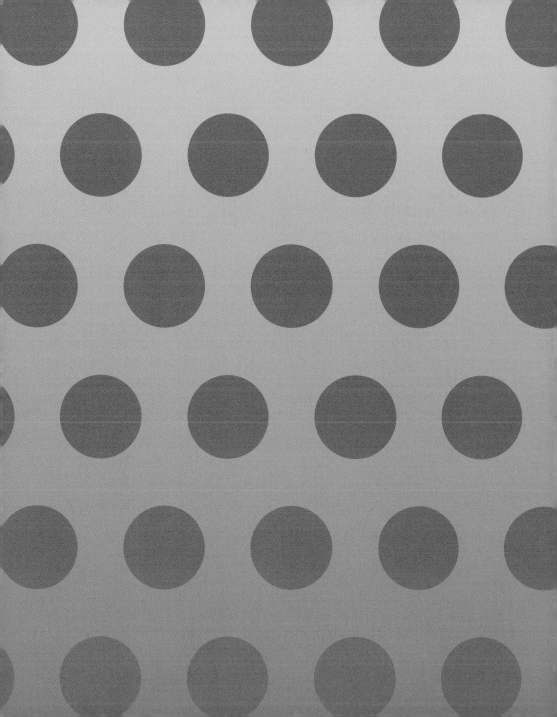

336. DOCTOR KNOWS BEST

If you suffer from any physical conditions or have had injuries in the past, consult your doctor before embarking on a fitness programme. Your doctor may have actually been the one to advise you to get fit in the first place. If that's the case, just get moving!

337. NEVER TOO LATE

People of all ages can benefit from exercise, so never think that you're too old (or young!) to start getting in shape. Late starters may find it a little tougher after years of sitting on the fence, but following a sensible routine can only lead you down one road – a healthier one.

338. LEARN THE TERMS

- Aerobic exercise provides an all-body workout that will improve heart health and burn fat. Aerobic exercises can be high impact (like jogging and star jumps), low impact (walking or cycling) or no impact (swimming). Greater impact means greater stress on your body.
- Anaerobic exercise is strength or resistance training. You use your muscles against weights or opposing forces (resistance). Not just for body-builders, this type of exercise tones and shapes muscles, and can be used to treat back pain.

339. WALK BEFORE YOU RUN

Set realistic goals for yourself. Think about what you want to achieve and shape your fitness programme around this. At first you might just want to improve your fitness levels and lose some weight. The fitness bug will bite, though, and you'll soon be more interested in toning certain areas of your body with resistance exercises (using weights).

340. HOW DOES YOUR HEART RATE?

Working towards a target heart rate will ensure you are exercising at a comfortable level. Beginners should aim for 50 per cent of their maximum heart rate, gradually working up to 85 per cent. To calculate your maximum heart rate, subtract your age from 220. For a 40 year-old, this would be 180 beats per minute (bpm). Fifty per cent of this is 90 bpm, so aim for that at first. Most gym machines will measure your heart rate, or you can buy a heart rate monitor.

341. PUTTING THE WHEELS IN MOTION

In the beginning, try to do at least 30 minutes of aerobic exercise (walking, jogging, swimming, cycling, aerobics or dancing) three or four times a week. Exercise shouldn't be a chore, so do something you enjoy. If you can only manage 15 minutes on some days, that's still better than doing nothing.

342. GOING FOR GOLD

Make a note of your fitness goals, making sure they are realistic and you know how to go about reaching them. If your goal is to lose weight, you'll need to combine a healthy-eating programme with your exercise plan.

343. WHERE DID THE DAY GO?

If you've planned to include 30 minutes of exercise in your day but find that you never quite get time to fit it in, split the 30 minutes into three (i.e. three sets of 10 minutes each). Ten minutes when you wake up, another 10 minutes at lunchtime and 10 minutes in the evening will fit much better into your routine – and it's not as daunting, either!

344. GET FIT FOR FREE

Take the stairs instead of the lift, walk up a moving escalator, park your car at the far end of the car park and hide the remote control so you have to get up to change television channels. Look for the difficult way to do things rather than taking the lazy way out.

345. GYM'LL FIX IT

Things to consider before joining a gym:

- location – should be near work or home
- opening hours – can you go when it suits you?
- staff – should be trained, experienced, helpful and approachable
- equipment – are there enough machines and a good selection?
- general maintenance – cleanliness, good lighting and ventilation
- pool – not all gyms have a pool, so consider its importance for you
- classes – a good option for people who need more motivation
- fees – shop around for the best deals

346. SPREAD YOUR ENTHUSIASM

You've joined a gym and bought new sports gear. You train most days for a month, and by the end of it, you're sore, tired and bored. To prevent yourself from going down this road to nowhere, begin slowly and build up gradually. Walk before running – literally!

347. PAY ATTENTION

Listen carefully during your gym induction so you know what machines you're using and why you're using them. Use the preset exercise programmes on the cardiovascular machines instead of relying on your own willpower to keep going. Read a fitness book or magazine for a better understanding of the different machines' uses.

348. KIT AND CABOODLE

Buy a nice sports bag and keep it equipped for gym visits. Include the following:

- water
- membership card
- workout clothes and footwear
- sweatband, hair ties
- towel – one for use during your workout and one for showering
- toiletries
- personal music system
- pedometer or heart rate monitor (optional)
- change of clothes (to wear after your workout, if necessary)

349. GOOD GYM ETIQUETTE

Here are some dos and some definite don'ts for gym visits:

- Dress appropriately – you might be proud of your abdominals, but not everyone wants to see them.
- Wipe down equipment after use.
- Don't spend too long on one piece of equipment at busy times. Most gyms will ask you to limit sessions to 20 minutes during peak times.
- Don't play your music too loudly, even if you have headphones – others can still hear it. And don't sing out loud!
- Keep grunting noises to yourself – this can be very off-putting to other gym members.
- Ask staff for help when you are using unfamiliar equipment, or if you injure yourself.

350. WARMING UP

Warming up and stretching before your workout will maximize results, help you enjoy the workout more and, most importantly, prevent injury. A good warm-up raises the body and muscle temperatures, and prepares your body for the demands of exercise by slowly increasing the blood circulation.

351. MARCHING ORDERS

For an easy, 10-minute warm-up on the spot, stand up straight, tucking in your behind and contracting your abdominals (the muscles that start under your chest and run down to just below your navel). Keep your chest up, with your shoulders held back. Bend your arms at the elbows until they are at a 90-degree angle in front of you. March on the spot at a slow pace, lifting your knees and pumping your arms up and down to get your heart rate up.

352. BEND AND STRETCH

Stretching should also form part of your warm-up.

- For shoulders, link your hands behind your back and extend your elbows. Slowly raise your arms as high as they will go without pain. Hold for 20 seconds.
- For hamstrings (the three muscles at the back of each thigh), stand with your right leg extended in front of you. It should be straight, with your left leg bent, supporting your weight. Bend forward slightly, keeping your back straight and your abdominals held tight. You should feel a stretch in the rear leg area. Hold for 15 seconds and switch legs.

353. AT A STRETCH

- For quadriceps (the four muscles at the front of each thigh), bend your right leg at the knee until your right foot almost touches your bum. Hold your foot in place with your right hand and slowly pull your foot in closer to your bum. Hold for 15 seconds, then repeat with your left leg.
- To stretch calves, place your hands against a wall. Extend one leg in front of you and one leg behind you. Bend the front knee, keeping the rear leg straight. Maintain this position during the stretch. Using your rear leg, push yourself towards the wall. Hold for 30 seconds, then change legs.

354. GETTING PERSONAL

Enlist the help of a personal trainer, at least initially, to set you on the right track to fitness. Most gyms offer this service, or you could check your phone book for freelance trainers. A personal trainer will assess your basic fitness level and recommend the best course of action for you to take in relation to your requirements.

355. SIMPLY THE BEST

There's no such thing as the best exercise or the best way to work out – nor is there a best time of day to exercise. It's up to you to establish what suits you and when it suits you best to exercise. Your body will adapt to your fitness routine after a few weeks, so do vary your workout occasionally.

356. ACCIDENTAL EXERCISE

If you're juggling work and family, there's no need to spend an hour a day at the gym to get your aerobic exercise. Walking instead of taking the car, climbing stairs instead of taking the lift, housework and cutting the lawn will all produce results.

357. BUDDY UP

Studies have shown that people with a fitness partner are more successful than those who go it alone. Companionship will motivate you, and making a commitment to another person will strengthen your commitment to your own fitness.

358. WALKIE TALKIE

You should be able to carry on a conversation during your workout. If you are breathless or can't talk you're working too hard, so slow down. Dizziness and feeling light headed are warning signs that you are overexerting yourself. If you experience either of these symptoms, stop your exercise and cool down.

359. TEAM WORK

If you're interested in joining a team to play sports, check out the different clubs in your area and go along for a trial to see what you think. They'll be delighted to have some fresh legs, so have a look in your phone book to see what you fancy.

360. WALK THIS WAY

Walking is one of the most popular exercises. It requires no special equipment other than a good pair of shoes. To maximize your workout, swing your arms, choose a challenging route with some hills and lengthen your strides.

361. PEDOMETER POWER

Invest in a pedometer – a small gadget that you clip onto your belt that will tell you how many steps you take. Aim for 10,000 steps each day and you'll find yourself making an extra effort to reach your target. Some pedometers will also calculate the number of calories you've burned once you've programmed it with your details.

362. PLODDING ALONG

Never walk with arm or ankle weights. They will damage your joints, leaving you at risk of injury. If you want to vary your walking workout, choose routes with some hills, increase the distance you cover or jog at intervals instead of walking all the time.

363. HOME GYM

Reasons to work out at home
- suits your schedule
- no peer pressure
- saves money
- doesn't depend on weather
- private and convenient

364. WINTER WORKOUT

Exposure to natural light boosts energy levels, relieves stress, regulates sleep patterns and improves overall mood. Try to get outdoors for at least 10 minutes each day in winter. Inhale plenty of fresh air – your lungs and skin will thank you after being subjected to air-conditioning and central heating for so long.

365. BABY, IT'S COLD OUTSIDE

Running outside on a cold day will burn more calories than running inside on a treadmill, or outside during the summer. Your body has to work harder in the cold weather to stay warm, so you'll use up more energy. Wrap up well and don't run when temperatures are below freezing.

366. CONCRETE INFORMATION
If you're running outside, avoid concrete surfaces, as they put pressure on your joints. Run on softer surfaces such as sand to strengthen your legs without damaging them.

367. TREAD CAREFULLY
When you're using a treadmill, start slowly and build up your speed at a gradual pace. Experiment with the incline but bear in mind that an incline of more than 10 per cent may strain your back and legs. Take normal strides but hold onto the rails at first if you need to. Pay attention to where you are on the treadmill so you don't fall back.

368. GET YOUR SKATES ON
An hour of ice-skating, roller-skating or rollerblading burns nearly as many calories as an hour of running, as well as strengthening ankle, knee and hip muscles. Ski machines in the gym have a similar effect, mimicking the motion of cross-country skiing to exercise arms and legs.

369. HOP, SKIP, JUMP
Skipping is not just for kids! It is a fantastic, cheap and easy way to get fit, providing a cardiovascular workout and improving endurance and coordination. Make sure the rope is the right length by stepping on the centre of the rope and bringing both handles upwards; they should reach chest height. For variation, elevate your knees while you are skipping and try different speeds.

370. IN THE SWIM
Swimming and aqua aerobics offer both aerobic and anaerobic workouts (see tip 338). The water provides resistance, helping you build muscle strength while improving your endurance and flexibility. You'll also get a cardiovascular workout and burn fat. It's never too late to learn to swim. Enquire about lessons at your local pool.

371. UPPER CLASS
In every town and city, you'll find a range of instructor-led classes like spinning, kick boxing and step aerobics, to name but a few. If you feel that you need more motivation to work out, this is a good option. Try a few different classes to see what you like. Committing to a prepaid term should help you go the distance.

372. LET'S DANCE
Salsa dancing is a fun, sexy way for both men and women to keep fit. Not only will it burn calories, but you'll also impress your friends with your new moves on the dance floor. Start off with a beginner's class. You don't have to bring a partner, as there will be others without partners who will be willing to pair up with you.

373. FOOTBALL CRAZY
Gather some friends together and organize a regular kick-about. You could hire an indoor or outdoor pitch one night a week and get a bit of competition going. Alternatively, just head to your local park on Sunday mornings and join in with the hundreds of other people who will also be there getting in shape!

374. REV IT UP
Short bursts of high-intensity training during your workout can boost your metabolism and improve your level of fitness. So, for example, if you're walking on the treadmill, increase the speed to a running level that's comfortable for you for 1 minute out of every 5 minutes.

375. TREAT YOUR FEET
Wear appropriate footwear for the exercise you are doing, with socks made from cotton to allow your feet to breath. Replace your trainers every 650 km (400 miles), or approximately every six months.

376. PENNYWISE
If you're thinking of investing in some gym equipment for a home gym, do your research. Consider durability, safety and added features that will hold your interest. Shop around and try before you buy. Consider how much room you have at home for the equipment and check that anything you buy has a warranty.

377. EXTRA VISION
Fitness DVDs and videos are a great way to get fit at home. Look for ones that offer three basic workouts – aerobic, resistance and flexibility. Select a level of training that suits you and don't feel that you have to follow at the same pace. The pause button is there for a reason, so use it if you need to!

378. STRETCHING THE TRUTH
Resistance bands are an affordable way to add variety to a workout. They come in varying degrees of resistance, with the more elastic ones offering less resistance. You can even practise your golf swing with them!

379. STAIR MASTER
Always take the stairs when you can. Stair climbing is more intensive than walking, because you lift your own body weight. Just 5 minutes of stair climbing each day can reduce your risk of heart disease and help prevent brittle bones.

380. CARRY ON CYCLING
Cycling is one of the best ways to exercise your cardiovascular system and burn calories. It strengthens your thighs, hips and buttocks without straining your muscles or joints. Always wear a helmet when you're cycling outdoors.

381. HOLE IN ONE
If you have time to spare at weekends and some money saved for a rainy day, take a few golf lessons. If you enjoy it, invest in a set of clubs and find a friend to join you on your rounds. You don't need to be a member of a golf club, and carrying your clubs around for two hours could help you burn 400 calories. Don't cheat with a golf buggy!

382. VACUUM WITH VIGOUR
Have a vigorous cardiovascular workout with the vacuum cleaner, squeeze your buttocks to tone them when you're ironing and clean your windows with both hands to strengthen your arms and shoulders.

383. 10-MINUTE TONING
Burn calories with 10 minutes of the following activities:
- housework – 35 calories
- cycling (medium pace) – 79 calories
- gardening – 58 calories
- ironing – 20 calories
- skipping – 93 calories
- yoga – 47 calories

384. THAT'S ENTERTAINMENT
Bring your own music to the gym, including plenty of upbeat tunes that inspire you and match your exercise pace. Working out should be fun and relaxing, not a boring chore.

385. KEEP IT IN THE FAMILY

If you have children who are on holiday from school, keep them entertained by planning outdoor activities like a trip to the beach, park or forest; a game of football; or a bike ride, so you can benefit from the activity, too.

386. HAPPY HOLIDAYS

The world is your oyster, so get out there and see it. Whether it involves cycling, hiking or sailing, an adventure holiday in the great outdoors will improve your level of fitness and get your adrenalin pumping. You might even save some cash!

387. GARDENING LEAVE

An hour of gardening can burn at least 300 calories per hour. It will also relieve stress and may even reduce your blood pressure. Work at a steady speed and change position every few hours. Use both sides of your body – pull up weeds with both hands rather than just one.

388. FLY YOUR KITE

Buy a kite (or make one), pack a picnic and take the family out for a fun-packed day. You'll be surprised at how much energy you will use up getting the kite airborne, keeping it in the air and, of course, untangling it when it falls! Beaches and hilltops are ideal for kite-flying.

389. GO THE EXTRA MILE

Ignore the calorie counter on workout machines. Unless they've been programmed with your details, the reading will be inaccurate. Think in terms of distance instead. Set yourself targets in kilometres or miles. It will feel good to leave the gym having cycled 10km (6 miles) and walked 5km (3 miles) in an hour.

390. EXERCISE CAUTION

Heed the following signs that you may be overdoing it:
- headaches or dizziness
- sore muscles
- decreased performance
- loss of appetite
- recurring illness or infection

391. STRESSED OUT

Drinking alcohol should be avoided when you are stressed. If you've had a hard day at work, don't head to the nearest pub to drown your sorrows. Do some exercise instead, and by the time you've finished, you'll have forgotten your work-related woes.

392. NO SWEAT

Fat is not lost in sweat, so don't worry if you don't seem to sweat as much as the person beside you. Concentrate on doing the exercises properly and drink plenty of water to replace the water that you lose when you do sweat.

393. FUELLING UP

Plan your eating around your activity:
- If you exercise early in the morning, have a light breakfast of some wholegrain toast or a small bowl of cereal before setting out.
- Wait at least an hour after a main meal before exercising.
- Drink plenty of water during and after exercise.
- Eat a light snack within half an hour of exercising. A banana, cereal or yoghurt are good choices.

394. MUSCLE IN ON CALORIE BURNING

Developing muscles, particularly your leg, chest, back and shoulder muscles, makes you burn more fat. Every 0.5kg (1lb 2oz) of muscle uses 50 calories to maintain itself. Defined muscles won't be visible if they are hidden by a layer of fat, though, so combine cardiovascular exercise with resistance training for optimum results.

395. WARM UP BEFORE WEIGHTS

Before you lift any weights, always warm up with some light cardiovascular activity, such as 10 minutes on the treadmill or exercise bike. This will help prevent muscle damage when you are toning, and you won't feel sore the following day.

396. WEIGHED DOWN

If you're toning up at home, you don't necessarily have to have dumb-bells or weights. Clasp some soup tins or heavy books in your hands, or partially fill a couple of 2-litre (3½-pint) bottles with sand or gravel. As you get stronger, you can increase the weight. A backpack filled with books will also provide resistance when you're walking or jogging – just make sure it's comfortable to carry.

397. BUILDING UP

Resistance-training exercises are measured in repetitions (reps) – the number of times you do each exercise. More repetitions with less resistance develops speed and stamina. Fewer repetitions and more resistance builds strength, power and size.

398. HEAVYWEIGHT

Using weights that are either too light or too heavy will affect your progress. As a rule of thumb, select a weight with which you can do eight or ten repetitions. If you can't finish eight, the weight is too heavy. If you can do ten easily, gradually increase the weight until you have found the right level.

399. QUALITY, NOT QUANTITY

You could do sit-ups until the cows come home and still not achieve a six-pack stomach. For toned abdominals, thighs and triceps (the muscles at the backs of your upper arms), you only need to do 15 to 20 repetitions of an exercise (about 10 minutes), two to three times a week. Concentrate on contracting the muscles in question and practise good breathing for success.

400. RESISTANCE RULES

The exercises that follow are intended to be done at home. You don't need any fancy equipment, although some exercises feature dumb-bells (see tip 396 for some household items you can use instead). Start with ten repetitions of each exercise. Don't use jerking movements and don't pull on your neck. Don't attempt any of these exercises if you have a history of back problems – consult your doctor for advice on suitable exercises.

401. SIX-PACK STOMACH

Lie on your back, with your knees bent and your feet flat on the floor. Put your hands behind your head for support. Concentrate on contracting your abdominals. Curl your shoulders upwards and forwards until your upper back lifts off the floor. Don't sit all the way up. Hold for 2 seconds, return slowly to your starting position, then repeat ten times.

402. TONE YOUR TRICEPS

Extend your left leg and bend it slightly. Place your left hand on your thigh for balance. Hold a weight in your right hand, with your elbow bent at a 90-degree angle at waist height. Without moving your upper arm, straighten your arm at the elbow so that the weight goes backwards. Repeat ten times, then switch sides.

403. BICEP CURLS

Hold your arms at your sides, with a weight in each hand and your palms facing your body. Align your elbows and wrists with your shoulders. Bend each arm at the elbow, while turning your wrists outwards until your palms are facing the ceiling. Lift the weights towards your shoulders without moving your upper arms. Stop the motion when the weights meet your shoulders; hold for one count. Return the weights to starting position. Repeat ten times.

404. BOTTOM LINE

While on your hands and knees, straighten your right leg, keeping your left leg bent to help support your weight. Slowly lift your right leg leg towards the ceiling, contracting your buttock muscles at the same time. Hold your leg at the top of the movement for one count. Lower your leg and repeat ten times. Change sides.

405. LUNGE AND SQUAT

Lunges and squats work your lower body and, combined with regular cardiovascular workouts, will shape and tone all areas of your legs, including your thighs, calves and bum.

406. LUNGES

Standing with your feet together, step forward with your right leg and lower your left leg, keeping both knees at 90-degree angles. Carrying the weight in your heels, push back up (slowly!) to starting position. Never lock your knees at the top and never let your right knee bend past your toes. Keep your upper body straight throughout the movement. Change sides and repeat ten times.

407. SQUATS

Standing with your feet shoulder-width apart, slowly lower your body as though you are going to sit in a chair, until your thighs are parallel to the ground. Keeping the weight in your heels, push yourself up slowly until you reach your starting position. Don't let your knees extend over your toes and don't slouch; keep your upper body straight! Change sides and repeat ten times.

408. FAX, PHONE, TONE

To tone your calf muscles at your desk, sit up straight with your feet around 30cm (12in) apart. Place the weight of your legs on the front or balls of your feet. Slowly lift your heels, toes still touching the floor, squeeze your calves, hold for one second and relax. Repeat ten times.

409. SPOT THE DIFFERENCE

If your thighs bother you, the bad news is that you won't be able to lose weight from that area alone because you can't spot-reduce fat. The good news is that through a healthy diet and exercise, you will be able to lose weight all over and reveal those shapely thighs.

410. TONE THOSE THIGHS

Sit on a chair with both of your feet on the floor. Extend your right leg straight in front of you. Point your toes upwards and squeeze your leg at the top of the movement. Hold for one second. Lower your leg to the ground. Repeat ten times, then switch to your left leg.

411. DECREASE YOUR DERRIÈRE

Lie on your back, with your knees bent, your feet flat on the floor and your arms by your side. Press your heels into the floor and gently lift your hips off the floor, squeezing your buttock muscles as you go. Breathe in, then lower and repeat ten times. Don't let your bum touch the ground between repetitions.

412. SWIM ON DRY LAND

This exercise works your lower back to strengthen it and prevent pain. Lie face-down on the floor with your arms and legs outstretched. Raise your left arm and your right leg a few centimetres (inches) off the floor. Lower and repeat with your right arm and left leg. Repeat ten times.

413. YOU'RE A STAR

Stand up straight with your chest and shoulders held back. Bend your arms at the elbows until they are at 90-degree angles. March on the spot, lifting your knees at a moderate pace for 3 minutes. Pump your arms up and down to increase your heart rate. Widen your stance and march for 30 seconds, keeping your knees slightly bent. Return to your starting position and march on the spot for the next minute. Now do ten star jumps.

414. STEP UP FOR GREAT LEGS

Stand facing a step, with your feet shoulder-width apart. Pushing off your right leg, step up with your left foot and follow with your right foot so that both feet are flat on the step. Step back down first with your left foot, then with your right, returning to your starting position. Repeat ten times.

415. SEATED LEG LIFT

Attach a leg weight (optional) to your right ankle. Sit on the floor, leaning back slightly and supporting your weight with your hands. Bend your left knee and keep your left foot on the floor. Slowly raise your right leg as high as you comfortably can. Repeat ten times, then swap to the left leg.

416. PUSH IT UP

Kneel on the floor, with your hands on the floor (palms facing down) and your arms and feet positioned slightly wider than shoulder-width apart. Straighten your back. Push your body up off the floor with your hands. Pause for a moment at the top of the movement. Exhale as you lower your body towards the floor, elbows coming out to the sides. Your chest should come within 5cm (2in) of the floor. Repeat ten times.

417. SHOULDER THE BLAME

To work your shoulders, sit up straight with your feet flat on the floor and your arms extended at your sides. Slowly circle your arms forwards, controlling the movements and focusing on your shoulder muscles. Do two sets of 12 repetitions, then change to backward circles.

418. GAINING WEIGHT

If you want to gain weight, you should maintain a healthy diet but increase your calorie intake by 500 calories. Lifting weights will build muscle, which also increases your weight. If you do these things but stop gaining weight, you will need to increase your calorie intake slightly.

419. TAKE A BREAK

It's not necessary to exercise every day of the week – but, at the same time, don't cram it all into one day. Spread your workouts over the week. Try doing cardiovascular and weight training on alternate days or, if you prefer, do both workouts on the same day, every second or third day, using the days in between as a rest period.

420. ON THE BALL

A fitness or Swiss ball is a bit like a giant beach ball and is great for toning and strengthening muscles. Study the instructions or ask a gym instructor how to use one properly and take care at first until you've learned how to balance. Just sitting on one to watch television can be a great challenge and will improve your posture.

421. BURN, BABY, BURN!

Try 30 minutes of the following activities and reap the rewards of calories burned!

- running at 16kmh/10mph – 525 calories
- playing football – 200 calories
- swimming – 315 calories
- basketball – 330 calories
- skipping – 279 calories
- squash – 308 calories
- cycling – 237 calories

422. PATIENCE IS A VIRTUE

Don't expect to see the beginnings of a six-pack stomach the day after your first crunch session. Losing weight and toning up takes time, and it might take up to eight weeks before you see the fruits of your labour. Don't lose heart – keep going and you will get there.

423. TAKE A HIKE!

Grab a partner or pack up the family and head to the hills for the day. Bring a picnic and plenty of water, and take in the scenery and fresh air around you. You probably see this scenery every day but just don't have time to appreciate it.

424. MAN'S BEST FRIEND

Feeling guilty about leaving your dog alone in the house all day? Walk him every evening to make up for it. Exercise helps animals live longer and keeps them more alert and content. Many behavioural problems like chewing, digging, and barking disappear once the animal engages in a regular activity.

425. BAREFOOT IN THE PARK

Yoga concentrates on a series of postures and breathing and relaxation techniques. It develops coordination and flexibility, as well as improving strength, balance and stamina. If yoga is new to you, join a beginners' class. You'll need comfortable clothes and a mat to lie on, but no special footwear as yoga is performed barefoot. Practice makes perfect, so once you know how to do the moves properly, run through them at home as often as possible.

426. YOGA TIME

If you're too busy to take a lunch break, take a few minutes to relax and stretch. Interlock your hands and raise your arms above your head. Turn your palms out towards the ceiling and gently lean to each side.

427. TOP FIVE WAYS TO BURN 100 CALORIES

- Play football for 15 minutes.
- Walk briskly for 16 minutes.
- Vacuum the house for 20 minutes.
- Walk up and down stairs for 10 minutes.
- Wash and polish the car for 20 minutes.

428. REVERSE YOUR ROUTE

Go in the opposite direction occasionally when you are jogging or walking. You'll climb and descend at different times, giving your muscles a new workout and offering you a change of scenery.

429. IN FITNESS AND IN HEALTH

Here's what not to do:
- Don't undertake a more intense activity than usual or exercise for longer periods than you're used to.
- Don't lift heavy weights if you haven't done so before.
- Don't ignore warning signs, like niggling pains, no matter how small they are.
- Don't exercise in extreme temperatures.
- Don't exercise if you're not feeling your best.

430. PILOT PILATES
Pilates is a series of controlled movements and is named after its founder, Joseph H. Pilates. It mainly focuses on abdominals and back muscles, so it can be good for toning, improving posture and strengthening back muscles for anyone prone to problems. Join a class and learn how to do the movements properly before practising them at home.

431. ANYONE FOR TENNIS?
Tennis is suitable for all ages and provides a great cardiovascular workout, as well as toning almost every muscle in the body. It also improves balance and coordination. One hour of singles tennis burns up to 550 calories, while a game of doubles could help you burn 400 calories.

432. FIRST AID
For most injuries, stop what you're doing and take an anti-inflammatory painkiller. Remember RICE: rest – take time out; ice – apply ice for up to 20 minutes (but do not do this more than twice in an hour); compression – wrap the injured area in an elastic bandage, but not too tightly; elevation – raise the injured body part to minimize swelling and help circulation. See a professional if the injury worsens or fails to get better.

433. OFF THE BEATEN TRACK

If you've had a break from your fitness routine, it can sometimes be hard to get back on track. Think about how much you enjoyed exercise before the break and the benefits you were reaping. Start slowly and you'll soon know how far you can push yourself.

434. WATER FEATURES

Drink plenty of water before, during and after exercise. The harder the workout, the more water you lose, so try to drink 300ml (12fl oz) every 15 to 20 minutes during your workout. Dehydration will set in if lost water isn't replaced, so don't wait until you're thirsty.

435. CORDIAL INVITE

There's no benefit to be gained from sports drinks. Despite their claims to replace lost electrolytes and keep you going for longer, most contain large amounts of sugar. Small amounts of sugar can enhance water absorption, but greater intakes cause bloating and cramps. Make yourself a healthier, less expensive drink by mixing a little low-sugar fruit cordial with your water.

436. COOL DOWN

Don't just stop exercising abruptly. Slow down towards the end of your workout and help your heart rate return to normal at a gradual pace. This will prevent you from feeling sick when you've finished. Some gentle stretches will relax your muscles, preventing soreness the next day.

WELL-
BEING

437. UNDER YOUR SKIN
Cellulite is a type of fat cell that gets trapped under your skin in groups. Unfortunately, there aren't any miracle treatments that will prevent it or help you get rid of it. Cellulite is worsened by poor diet, a sedentary lifestyle and poor circulation – so eliminate toxins by eating more healthily and starting an exercise programme, and incorporate some massage into your daily routine. Aim to drink at least 2 litres (3½ pints) of water a day.

438. LOOK ON THE BRIGHT SIDE
When you begin to eat better and exercise more regularly, you will find yourself feeling more optimistic about the changes you're making. Having a bright outlook keeps you motivated and moving forward – and inspires you to make more positive decisions!

439. MINI BREAK
Today's lifestyle is time-restricted and overloaded with information, and moves at such a fast pace that you get caught up in the race and lose sight of who you are and what you're trying to do. Take a few minutes during the day to pause and think about why you may feel out of sync or over-anxious, or why you're eating too much or exercising too little. Record this in a journal and continue refining and growing every day.

440. STUB IT OUT

If you're a smoker, it's time to seriously consider quitting. Look at the benefits to be gained:

- easier breathing
- increased energy levels
- healthier skin and nails
- increased chance of conceiving if you want to try for a baby
- cleaner, fresher clothes, house, car and hair
- food tastes better
- increased confidence
- healthier for all the family

441. KICKING THE HABIT

Don't go it alone if you're trying to quit smoking. Chat with your pharmacist about nicotine-replacement products and choose one that suits you. Don't use cigarettes as a crutch for stressful or emotional situations – they only provide temporary relief. If you're afraid of gaining weight, take it one step at a time. Concentrate on quitting smoking, then focus on your weight.

442. HAVE A MASSAGE

Massage is a popular technique that treats pain and encourages relaxation. In conventional medicine, it is widely used in sports treatments and physiotherapy, with plenty of research to support its use. In complementary medicine, it is used to treat pain, muscular discomfort, general ill health, anxiety, fatigue and depression.

443. RELAX AND SOOTHE
Add a few drops of rose aromatherapy oil to bathwater to help relieve stress, ease inflammation and soothe muscle tissues. It is also believed to cleanse your liver and encourage circulation.

444. EASE THE SNEEZE
If you suffer from hay fever but find that antihistamines don't agree with you, take grape seed extract in conjunction with vitamin C to relieve symptoms. Vitamin C is a natural antihistamine, and both supplements will boost your immunity.

445. ALLERGY PROOFING
Proof your home against hay fever and other allergy triggers during pollen season. Keep your bedroom windows and doors shut in mid-morning and early evening. Don't hang your clothes out to dry, as they will collect pollen. Keep dust to a minimum by vacuuming regularly and using a damp cloth for dusting.

446. MIND YOUR BACK!
Back pain is a major cause of disability, affecting millions of people each year. Protect your back when you are lifting and putting things down by always bending your knees instead of bending your back. Keep your feet apart for stability and hold the item that you are moving close to your body.

447. FINDING A BALANCE
Good balance will send the right messages to the brain and help prevent falls. Spend a few minutes each day practising good balance. Stand up straight, holding onto the back of a chair. Raise one leg slightly off the floor. Try to balance for 10 seconds, then repeat five times, alternating legs. As your balance improves, try to do this exercise without holding onto the chair.

448. TENSE TYPING
Keep your wrists, fingers and neck supple and healthy after long stretches at the computer with the following exercises. Repeat each one three times:
- Stretch your wrists backwards for a few seconds, then forwards.
- Spread your fingers apart, then make a fist. Hold for a moment and repeat.
- Tuck in your chin and slowly bend your neck forwards. Hold for a few seconds, then repeat.

449. FLY BY NIGHT
Preparation will make a long-haul flight more comfortable. Request a seat by the emergency exit, bring an eye mask to minimize disturbances and wear comfortable clothes with extra layers (or bring a small blanket) in case it's cold. Drink plenty of water and avoid alcohol. Walk or move around regularly to prevent deep vein thrombosis (DVT). Wearing flight socks has also been shown to reduce the risk of DVT.

450. LAGGING BEHIND
To avoid jet lag, go to bed a few hours earlier on the nights before your trip. Avoid alcohol during the flight and drink lots of water. Take some exercise when you arrive at your destination and spend time outside to get some natural light. Adjust your meal and sleeping times to your new time zone as soon as possible to help synchronize your body clock.

451. HEALTHY HOLIDAY
Always take out travel insurance. Check if you need extra vaccinations for your destination and organize them well in advance. Take a small first-aid kit and, if you take medication, carry enough with you to last the holiday, plus a little extra. Never drink water in a foreign country unless you are sure it is safe.

452. IMMOBILE
The jury is still out on the potential damage to health caused by mobile phones. However, it is well established that they can be a cause of stress, so switch yours off whenever possible. If you mostly use your phone for work, turn it off in the evenings and at weekends. Anyone who calls can leave a message!

453. LOVE YOURSELF
Low self-esteem stems from underlying issues and can lead to other problems, such as eating disorders, strain in your relationships and depression. Seek counselling to try to overcome the issues that are holding you back from being you; only by dealing with them can you learn to love yourself.

454. JOIN THE PARTY CIRCUIT
Surrounding yourself with close friends and family will help you enjoy a healthier life. Friends encourage people to look after their health and can reduce feelings of anxiety and depression whenever the going gets tough.

455. HOT STONES
Find a therapist or spa that offers a hot-stone massage for a soothing treatment. It helps relieve tension and stress, soothes injured or tired muscles and improves circulation.

456. ST JOHN'S WORTH IT?
St John's Wort is a herbal remedy that is mainly used to treat depression, anxiety, insomnia and stress. It can interfere with the effectiveness of prescribed medication, however, so before taking it, consult with your doctor to check if it is safe for you to use.

457. ECHINACEA
Echinacea, another herbal remedy, is largely used for its immunity-boosting properties in the treatment of colds. It is believed to have anti-inflammatory, antiseptic, antiviral, antibacterial and antiallergenic properties. Take it in tablet or droplet form at the first sign of a cold, but don't take it for more than two weeks at a time.

458. THE MORNING AFTER
Milk thistle is a herbal remedy that protects the liver and is sometimes used in the treatment of liver disorders. It is an effective hangover cure if you take it before you go to bed on the night of a heavy drinking session – or even just before you start to drink.

459. NIGHT FEVER
If you or your partner snores, it could prove to be detrimental to your relationship. Sleeping on your side rather than your back can prevent snoring. Quitting smoking and losing weight may help. Also consider burning some eucalyptus oil in your bedroom before you go to sleep.

460. SPOT CHECK
Acne can be treated with conventional medicine, but there are a few other things you can also do to treat it. Cleanse affected areas with tea tree oil, which has an antibacterial effect. Avoid touching the affected area with your hands and don't squeeze spots. This will prevent infection and scarring.

461. BATHE LIKE CLEOPATRA
Adding a few drops of coconut milk to your bathwater will revive and moisturize your skin, thanks to its oil content. Coconut milk is especially good for skin after you have spent a long winter indoors.

462. PRACTISE BODY BRUSHING
Buy a body brush and use it every day on dry skin before you shower. Brush up towards your heart, starting from the bottoms of your legs. Body brushing gets rid of dead skin cells, improves circulation, prevents cellulite and softens skin.

463. FAKING IT
Don't be tempted to use a sunbed. Far from giving you a healthy glow, it will give you freckles and brown skin – signs of damage – and increase your risk of developing skin cancer. Opt for fake tan to take away that milky-white appearance.

464. PERFECT PICNIC
Tea tree oil is a natural herbal remedy with antimicrobial, antiseptic, antifungal, insect-repellant and deodorizing properties. Pack it for the hazards – brambles, nettles, wasps and other insects – you might encounter on a country picnic.

465. FEELING THE PINCH
Bites and stings can be extremely painful and itchy, and if scratched the skin may become broken, risking infection. To ease symptoms, apply ice to the affected areas. Administer diluted lemon juice to wasp stings and a solution of ice-cold water mixed with bicarbonate of soda to bee stings. Vinegar also relieves any stinging, especially from sea creatures such as jelly fish.

466. LAUGHTER: THE BEST MEDICINE
Laughing boosts blood flow, and researchers say that 15 minutes of laughter a day as well as regular exercise could reduce your risk of cardiovascular disease. Laughing has previously been found to help fight infections, relieve hay fever, ease pain, lower stress levels and control breathing.

467. FUN IN THE SUN
Vitamin D is made through the action of sunshine on your skin – but this isn't a licence to bake yourself. Vitamin D can still be made through sunscreen, so slather on the factor 20 and choose a moisturizer with a sun-protection factor of at least 15 to prevent ageing.

468. FANCY FOOTWORK
Look after your feet to prevent corns, bunions and other problems. Wear shoes that fit properly and remove them whenever possible to allow your feet to breathe. Soaking your feet in a footbath of warm water and Epsom salts will soothe and soften hard skin.

469. UNDER THE KNIFE
If you are considering cosmetic surgery, check out the credentials and registration details of your chosen surgeon, hospital or clinic. Take a partner or friend to your first consultation, as there will be a lot of information to take in. Make sure you are well informed of any risks involved and the expected recovery times before proceeding.

470. PROTECT YOURSELF
If you've taken risks with your sexual health in the past, have a sexual health exam. Some sexually transmitted infections have no symptoms, so even if you feel fine, get yourself checked out.

471. DON'T LIVE TO WORK
Strike a healthy balance between work and 'you' time. Learn to switch off when you leave work. If you're unhappy in your job, it will spill over into your personal life, so try to identify why you're unhappy and try to resolve any problems.

472. TAKE A BREAK
Don't waste your days off with visits to the dentist or doctor – use your time off from work purposefully and imaginatively. Take advantage of cheap flights or last-minute holiday deals and really get away from it all.

473. DECLUTTER
Clutter can be tiring. You trip over it and spend time tidying it up, but it also makes you sigh when you see it. Don't tackle it all at once – set aside an hour each week, perhaps on a Sunday morning, to have a good clear out. This doesn't mean you have to get rid of your childhood teddy bear, but be realistic.

474. RECOGNIZE YOUR STRENGTHS
Most of us spend time concentrating on our weaknesses, rather than focusing on, and making the most of, our strengths. Write down what you believe to be your top ten strengths, and remind yourself of them when you're having a bad day.

475. SPA WELL

Recharge your batteries by checking into a hotel with a spa for a weekend break. Relax, have a massage and just enjoy being pampered. Yes, you, too, sir!

476. SLEEP EASY

- Don't eat a heavy meal or have caffeine-containing drinks before bedtime.
- Invest in a good-quality mattress and pillows.
- Keep your bedroom stress free; leave anything related to work in another room.
- Don't sleep with the television or bright lights on.

477. WEIGH UP THE ALTERNATIVES

Alternative therapies can offer a fresh approach to good health. Choose a qualified practitioner who is registered with the relevant professional body. Before embarking on a course of complementary medicine, talk it over with your doctor, especially if you take medication. Never change or stop taking medication unless advised by your doctor.

478. QUESTIONS TO ASK AN ALTERNATIVE THERAPIST

- Are you registered as a trained practitioner with a professional body?
- Are you qualified with a reputable educational or training organization?
- Are you experienced in treating conditions like mine?
- Are there any risks involved in treatment?
- How long will the treatment last?
- How much do you charge?

479. PINS AND NEEDLES
Acupuncture is an ancient Chinese therapy and one of the most thoroughly researched alternative medical practices. It works by stimulating your body's own healing responses and re-establishing any energy or 'chi' imbalances. Consider it for pain relief, stress, depression and reducing dependencies.

480. CLEAR THE WAY
Reflexology works on the principle that points on your feet represent energy pathways to different parts of your body. Blockages in these energy pathways are thought to lead to illness or imbalance. By working on particular points on your feet, a reflexologist aims to clear these blockages.

481. UNDER A SPELL
Hypnosis is a state of intense relaxation and concentration. Consider it to help you break bad habits such as smoking, or to relieve pain. Hypnosis will only happen if you want to be hypnotized, so you are in control of what happens.

482. AROMATHERAPY
Aromatherapy uses a range of essential plant oils to relax you, restore your emotional well-being, increase your energy levels and reduce stress. The oils are diluted and massaged into your skin. They can also be inhaled. Seek advice before using any essential oils yourself, especially if you are pregnant or have an illness. In their natural form, essential oils can irritate your skin.

483. HOMEOPATHY
Homeopathic remedies can help in the treatment of many illnesses and conditions, from hay fever to irritable bowel syndrome (IBS). It is based on the principle that symptoms are the body's defences and need to be encouraged to develop rather than being suppressed. A homeopath aims to find a remedy that in high doses produces symptoms similar to those of your condition. You then take this remedy in a diluted form.

484. CRUISING FOR A BRUISING
Arnica is a very effective homeopathic remedy for bruising. You can buy it in cream form to rub on the bruise or take it internally as soon as the bruising occurs. Keep applying the cream until the bruise begins to clear. Don't use arnica on open wounds.

485. WAKE UP TO WASTE
Unnecessary packaging on food is damaging to the environment, which in turn will have an impact on our health. Try to buy loose fruit and vegetables rather than pre-packed bags, and buy your meat, fish and poultry from the butcher's and fish counters instead of getting it in pre-packed trays. Cutting down on convenience foods in your diet will also reduce wasteful packaging.

486. HEALTH RECORDS
Keep a small diary with a record of any health-related visits to your doctor, dentist, specialist or the hospital – including a short note about the outcome of each visit. This will help you remember when to schedule subsequent visits and will remind you what the last one was about.

487. SKIN DEEP

Know your skin type and choose suitable moisturizing and cleansing products accordingly – this applies to you men out there, too! Oily skin tends to have open pores, a greasy appearance and is prone to spots. Dry skin feels tight and sometimes itchy after washing and may be flaky in some areas. Combination skin is usually oily around the forehead, nose and chin but dry in other areas.

488. TOP TEN FOODS FOR HEALTHY SKIN

- kiwi fruit
- avocados
- blackcurrants
- salmon
- green tea
- water
- yoghurt
- tomatoes
- oranges
- walnuts

489. ON THE SPOT

Don't pick at your spots – this will only cause scars to form. Also never touch your face with greasy hands, as this could clog up your pores. Dab a small amount of toothpaste on spots overnight and wash it off the next morning. This will dry out your spots and help them heal faster.

490. LIP SERVICE

Pay as much attention to your lips as you do to your skin. Exfoliate them gently with an old toothbrush to get rid of old, dry skin and use petroleum jelly to keep them soft and smooth. If you have a cold, put a little petroleum jelly around your nose to prevent it from becoming cracked and sore.

491. HARD AS NAILS

If you have dry hands, and your nails are weak and flaky, soak your hands in a small bowl of warm olive oil once a week. This will strengthen your nails and make your hands silky soft.

492. FLOSS IS THE BOSS

Floss your teeth regularly before brushing to loosen food particles, make your teeth cleaner and reduce the risk of tooth decay – floss reaches areas that your toothbrush can't. Wind a short length of waxed dental floss around the second finger on each hand and slide it down between your teeth. Gently remove the floss and repeat for all teeth.

493. MOUNTAINS AND MOLEHILLS

If you have moles on your body, regularly check them for changes in appearance. If you notice any that have changed colour, size or shape, or look different from your other moles, bring this to the attention of your doctor.

494. SEAWEED SPECIAL

Treat yourself to a seaweed bath. It's great for detoxing and will rehydrate and moisturize your skin – so it's especially good after a holiday in the sun. Seaweed baths can also relieve conditions like acne, eczema, back pain and arthritis, as well as helping speed up wound healing.

495. RAW EGGS

Avoid eating raw eggs if you are pregnant, unwell or elderly, and don't give them to children under five years of age. Raw eggs carry the risk of salmonella, which is a type of food poisoning. Foods that may contain raw eggs include tiramisu, mayonnaise and ice-cream, so if you are eating out, ask about ingredients.

496. HEADING SOUTH

Ladies should invest in a good sports bra for exercising. Insufficient support could strain or damage fragile tissues and cause pain. A well-fitting sports bra will prevent this.

497. WAX LYRICAL

Try Hopi ear candling to relieve sinus problems, compacted ear wax, headaches, colds and hay fever. Performed by a qualified therapist using special tubes filled with beeswax and honey, it draws impurities out of your ear and relieves congestion, while at the same time relaxing you.

498. HAIR RAISING

If your hair is looking dull and lifeless, or feeling dry and brittle, it could be a sign that your diet is lacking in something. Hair problems often indicate an insufficient intake of calories or protein. If your eating habits have been erratic, try to include plenty of lean protein such as chicken and fish, or plant-based protein foods like quinoa, beans and pulses, in your diet.

499. BODY ODOUR

Everybody perspires, especially in hot weather, but apart from wearing anti-perspirant, there are certain foods you can avoid to minimize body odour. These include garlic, onions, strong-smelling spices and asparagus. Drinking sage tea helps reduce sweating and is especially good if you experience menopausal sweating and hot flushes.

500. BETTER SAFE THAN SORRY

Even if there is a good health service available to you, it's a good idea to have health insurance. This will give you peace of mind if you ever need any kind of treatment for which you wish to go private rather than joining a long waiting list.

501. AND FINALLY . . .

Once again – drink water! The importance of drinking water for good health really can't be emphasized enough. Hopefully, after mentioning water in every chapter of this book, I've convinced you to drink 2 litres (3½ pints) of water each day. It's the easiest and most effective health tip of all!

Glossary

BAD (LDL) CHOLESTEROL
Low density lipoprotein cholesterol, also known as 'bad' cholesterol, provides essential cholesterol in the body, but too much can lead to blockage of the arteries and the formation of plaques that could cause heart disease and stroke.

CALORIES
The energy we use to live is measured in calories or kilocalories (the two terms mean the same thing). The number of calories you need depends on your age, gender, activity level and size, among other things. Energy is also measured in kilojoules. 1 kilocalorie = 4.18 kilojoule.

CARDIOVASCULAR WORKOUT
Cardiovascular exercise like cycling, swimming or running can improve heart and lung health, increase circulation and help with weight loss.

CELLULITE
Cellulite is an accumulation of fatty deposits underneath the skin, resulting in a dimpled, uneven appearance. It usually appears around the thighs or buttocks.

COMPLEX CARBOHYDRATE
Complex carbohydrates are composed of starch and fibre, and are found in plant foods such as breakfast cereal, bread, pasta, rice and some vegetables. The World Health Organisation (WHO) recommends that at least 50 per cent of the calories in your diet should come from complex carbohydrates.

ESSENTIAL FATTY ACID
Essential fatty acids are fats that we must obtain from our diets because they can't be made in the body. They are also known as linoleic acid (often called Omega 6) and linolenic acid (often called Omega 3).

EXTRINSIC SUGAR
Extrinsic sugars are sugars that are usually added to foods during manufacturing, and are not found naturally in those foods. Examples include table sugar, fruit squashes, cakes and biscuits. Lactose in milk is an extrinsic sugar, but for nutritional purposes it is not grouped with other extrinsic sugars.

FREE RADICAL
A free radical is an unstable molecule in the body that can damage cells and accelerate the progression of cancer, heart disease and ageing.

GLUCOSAMINE
Glucosamine is made in the body and is a major component of cartilage. Glucosamine supplements are often advised for sufferers of arthritis as they can help repair damaged arthritic joints and reduce pain.

GOOD (HDL) CHOLESTEROL
High density lipoprotein cholesterol, also known as 'good' cholesterol, is believed to help prevent blockage of the arteries and therefore reduce the risk of heart disease.

INSOLUBLE FIBRE
Insoluble fibre is a type of fibre made from cellulose and is mainly found in plant foods. Good sources include vegetables, pulses, beans and rice. An adequate intake of insoluble fibre is important for preventing constipation.

INSULIN
Insulin is a hormone made in the body by the pancreas. The body's cells need it to break down glucose for energy.

INTRINSIC SUGAR
Intrinsic sugars are found naturally in foods; they are part of the cellular structure of foods such as fruit and vegetables.

MONOUNSATURATED FAT

Monounsaturated fats are usually liquid at room temperature. They are believed to help lower levels of bad (LDL) cholesterol and increase levels of good (HDL) cholesterol in the body, thereby reducing the risk of heart disease and some cancers. Monounsaturated fats are found in greatest quantities in olive oil, rapeseed oil, nuts, avocados and olives.

MUSCLE GROUPS

- abdominals (abs) – under the chest down to just below the navel
- biceps – front of upper arms; used for lifting light objects
- deltoids (delts) – shoulders, tops of arms
- gluteus maximus (glutes) – 'buns' or buttock muscles; largest in the body
- hamstrings – three muscles at the back of each thigh
- lats – from below shoulders to lower back; largest back muscle
- pectorals (pecs) – chest muscles
- quadriceps (quads) – four muscles at the front of each thigh
- trapezius (traps) – from neck to shoulders and down centre of back
- triceps – back of upper arms; used when you're pushing something (e.g. a pram, a lawnmower or a shopping trolley)

OXIDATION

Oxidation is a chemical reaction that occurs when a substance combines with oxygen. Free radicals can cause oxidation in the body and, as a result, damage cells.

PHYTOCHEMICAL

Phytochemicals are chemicals found naturally in plant foods. They are thought to promote good health, boost immunity and decrease the risk of diseases such as cancer.

PHYTONUTRIENT

Phytonutrients are similar to phytochemicals. They are found in plant foods such as fruit, vegetables and wholegrains, and their effects on health are similar to those of phytochemicals.

POLYUNSATURATED FAT

Polyunsaturated fat is a type of fat contained in vegetable oils such as corn oil, sunflower oil and walnut oil. It is believed to help lower levels of bad (LDL) cholesterol in the body.

PREBIOTICS AND PROBIOTICS

Prebiotics nourish the bacteria that are already present in the digestive system. They often go hand in hand with probiotics as they create a hospitable atmosphere in the gut in which probiotic bacteria can grow and thrive. The most common prebiotic, inulin, is found in garlic, onions, artichokes, bananas and wholegrains. Probiotics are naturally occurring, live bacteria that are added to some foods to replenish levels of good bacteria that occur naturally in the gut. Specific strains of probiotic bacteria, such as L. acidophilus, L. casei and B. bifidus, can prevent the growth of 'unfriendly' bacteria in the gut.

REFINED CARBOHYDRATE

Refined carbohydrates are foods that have been processed by machinery to remove the high fibre constituents (bran and germ) from the grain. Examples include white flour, pasta, sugary breakfast cereals and white rice.

SATURATED FAT

Saturated fat is usually solid at room temperature and is mainly found in animal products such as butter, cream, meat and eggs. It can raise levels of bad (LDL) cholesterol in the body, and diets high in saturated fat have been linked with health problems such as obesity and heart disease.

SOLUBLE FIBRE

Soluble fibre dissolves in the gut and forms a gel that can slow down the release of sugar and nutrients from food. It can therefore help control blood sugar levels and also reduce the risk of heart disease by lowering levels of bad (LDL) cholesterol in the body. Soluble fibre is mainly found in apples, citrus fruits, oats, barley, rye and pulses.

TRANS FAT

A trans fat is an unsaturated fat that has been altered during processing – for example, converting vegetable oil to margarine. Trans fats are similar to saturated fats but may be more damaging than saturated fats; not only do they increase levels of bad (LDL) cholesterol but they may also reduce levels of good (HDL) cholesterol. Trans fats are found in margarines, take-away foods and baked goods like cakes and biscuits.

UNIT (OF ALCOHOL)

A unit of alcohol is 10 ml (0.5fl oz) of pure alcohol.
The following measures all contain one unit of alcohol:

- a glass of wine – 100 ml (3½fl oz)
- approximately half a pint of beer, lager or cider – 220 ml (8fl oz)
- a 25-ml (1-fl oz) measure of spirits

Index